WILL I MAKE IT?

AN AUTOBIOGRAPHY
of
WHAT IT'S LIKE LIVING WITH EPILEPSY
BY

ROBERT POSL

ISBN: 1542347173
ISBN-13: 978-1542347174

DEDICATION

This book is dedicated to every doctor, neurologist, specialist, or in other words practically anybody, who works in the field of neurology, especially epilepsy, making the lives and futures of people suffering from epilepsy, or any neurological condition, that much easier and better.

ACKNOWLEDGMENTS

There are obviously many people who have been by my side, as I pushed forward along the road of life. But there are certain individuals who played a unique part in my life during this time, living with epilepsy and in writing my story:

First and foremost, I would especially like to thank my neurologist, Dr. Bogdan Lorber. He is my neurologist and he covered my condition almost from the beginning. He didn't just carry out his basic obligations as my neurologist; prescribing my medications and cover the basics of treating my condition - as most doctors do. Dr. Lorber also takes time to speak with me, the patient and answers any questions I may have about my condition. Even when we meet outside of the doctor's room, he takes the time to show interest in my wellbeing.
It was through consultations with him, that my interest in epilepsy actually originated and grew, because he gave me the feeling that I myself can think about, and also do something about, the condition.

I would also like to thank the writer Noah Charney, who encouraged me to start writing. He helped me stay confident and 'strong' as I was writing; giving me advice, words of assistance about writing and so on. Just listening to him and what he has to say as a writer is always encouraging and often interesting.

You know how people often say, “The day started off quite normally,” Well, don’t they always? That was how it was for me on the 10’th of July 1994, when I went hiking with my cousin and his wife.
But the day didn't end up as it normally would, or as it should have. But far from that, and far from what anybody would want. The events of that day were destined to add to a number of events which were going to make 1994 a year of my life with great changes and detours. More than anybody could ever imagine. Changes which were destined to detour life down entirely different roads than it otherwise would have taken.

It all started more or less in the second half of 1993, when the idea of moving to Slovenia first came to light. Up until then I had lived quite a discreet life, with nothing really special to note.

I have always had an interest and curiosity in writing. The use of the English language never was my speciality though, but as the idea and encouragements to write my story mounted, I started writing. But it wasn’t until I started showing some of my notes to a therapist involved in the rehabilitation of patients after traumatic experience and the reactions and replies I got from him, that I saw the advantages and benefits of sharing my story, that it became something I was determined to see to the end.

Chapter one

As a child I was somewhat more on the shy side. I didn't have much of self-esteem either, which was often and easily 'run over' by the ego and domination of my schoolmates. I lived quite a discrete life, not socialising or mingling with other peers much at all. But as I grew up, so did my self-worth and my self-esteem. This was especially evident in the transition from primary school to high-school. This transition was quite a big one for me, since it was a period in my life when I also started finding some direction in life. It was as if I was slowly coming out from under the rock I had been hiding under.

This growth in my self-esteem was evident practically everywhere. I became your typical Highveld boy, growing up and enjoying the freedom of the open air of the South African Highveld. This was the backbone of the person I was to become, as someone who enjoys the freedom of outdoors. I enjoyed spending my free time either alone or with my friends from school, spending more and more time out and about under the baking African sun, rather than just at home and with the neighbouring kids. My life in general had started to widen out.

Another introduction, or rather change was that when I started going to high school, new and more interesting subjects made going to school actually quite interesting. This growth and change was especially evident in my results at school, as well as in my extra-curricular activities.

In the first year of high-school, I joined the athletics team and became quite active and actually quite successful in that. My participation in athletics endured almost all the way to the end of high-school.

The same was true for my achievements at school. As soon as I started with more technical subjects, I began receiving awards for my achievements there, which also continued all the way into my final year at high-school.

While I was at high-school, there were quite a lot of changes happening in the world in general. Some of which were directly associated with our family and family life.

The first change was that in 1991, Slovenia broke away from the former communist country of Yugoslavia. This change made travelling to and from Slovenia so much easier than it used to be, since obtaining a visa, or in other words permission to enter or leave the country, was now a walk in the park compared to what it had been before. It was as if Slovenia too had crawled out from under its hiding place, as I did with my transition.

I started hearing more about and slowly got to know relatives I had never seen or even heard of before. The first greater event was when my uncle and his wife came to visit us in South Africa. This was the start of more frequent movement to and from Slovenia, the country from where my parents originated.

But now the future for Slovenia was looking quite promising, since it was now coming out of the dark and getting that much closer to becoming a European state.

Other big changes happening almost at the same time, were the goings-on of the political situation in South Africa. It was clear that the apartheid era, which was so dominant in South Africa in the 1970's and 80's, was coming to an end. Thus, the future for South Africa was looking rather unsure. South Africa was bound to follow in the footsteps of Rhodesia before it, or worse, is what most feared and predicted. Thus, the chances of being able to create and have a successful, constructive future and life in South Africa didn't look good at all, and many wanted to immigrate.

As a result of all these changes and goings on, my parents started making more visits to Slovenia. Up until then, neither of them had ever been back. And us, as children who had obviously never been to Slovenia, or Yugoslavia as it was before. We were now hearing so much more about it. We were slowly but surely getting to know the country from where my parents originated.

As time went on, the idea and option of moving back to Slovenia became ever more tempting and real. It became quite a regular topic around the dinner table. With time, it became quite a realistic idea, since the prospect of a pleasant life in South Africa was looking ever grimmer, while almost the opposite was happening in Slovenia.

All this was happening as I was progressing towards the end of my high-school years. By the time I eventually reached the final year, and thus the last few months of high school, the decision to emigrate had all-but been made. If I was going to emigrate, this was going to be the ideal time to do it; I was completing with high-school and had not yet applied or signed up for any course at any university.

It was actually just before I even finished with high-school that my father made a visit to Slovenia. It was during that visit that he enquired if it would be possible for me to apply for a course at a university in Slovenia with my high-school certificate from South Africa. The news he brought back home made it almost a confirmation. I was going to move to Slovenia.

Well, there you go, my parents were going to end up where they started, almost 35 years before. But in an entirely different country. I was glad that my parents took on this great circle, this great life adventure. We might have ended up back in the country from where my parents originated, but we are for surely enriched by all we have experienced and picked up on the way.

Looking back at it all, I see that I am much richer than most people around me...

Chapter two

I successfully and with honours graduated from high-school. The time after graduation was initially laid back and easy going, with almost no obligations, tasks or anything really to worry about. But as time went on, and as the date of my move to Slovenia came ever so much closer, the reality of what was about to happen started to dawn on me.

Being barely twenty years old, I don't think I fully realized what I was getting in to, or what I was about to do. I was preparing to leave home, leave my parents, leave the surroundings I grew up in and was so familiar with, and move to another continent.

That was it, with a suitcase in one hand and my packed bike in the other I left home, South Africa and headed off for Europe. This was the first of a couple of events that were going to make 1994 a year with events and changes, which were going to entirely change me and my life as I knew it.

I arrived in Slovenia for the very first time on the 14'th of June 1994. I met relatives I had never met before and was going to get a lot more acquainted with the new surroundings where I was going to spend the next few years of my life. I met the relatives I was going to live with already in the first few days after arriving in Slovenia. I also, you could say, 'met' the place and surroundings where I was going to live. My relatives live in a village with a beautiful view of the Slovenian Alps.

One of the beauties and great attractions of Slovenia are its mountains. For many, hiking in the Slovenian Alps is an obvious 'must-do' to experience.

That is how it was with the relatives I was going to live with. They are keen hikers and enjoy the outdoors. It didn't take long before they had planned and organised a hike in the nearby mountains. It was the middle of summer, the weather was ideal, and the route not too challenging. Ideal for somebody like myself, who is not an experienced hiker.

The hike into the mountains was all going well and according to plan, until, that is, we began to descend. We were more than halfway down the mountainside, where it was more comfortable and easier walking. Then it happened! I tripped and fell onto the rocks. I injured myself pretty badly. My cousin's wife, who was with us, ran back up the mountain to call for help. That was it. I don't remember the rest, except for a couple of words spoken by one of the rescue team and the noise of the helicopter, as we flew out of the mountains towards the city. That was the second significant event which was destined to make 1994 a year of change for me and for my life.

I woke up a week later in hospital. My recovery and rehabilitation went well and quite quickly too. Life returned to normal. Well, at least in terms of my health, and with regards to what had happened to me it did. I was back at home with my relatives, learning a new language and meeting new people.

I was also preparing for the start of classes at the university in Ljubljana, the capital of Slovenia. So, life was quite hectic and what many would consider, 'far from normal'.

Two months later I started attending classes at the university. Up until then I had spent practically all my time with relatives. But now I was meeting all kinds of people, from different backgrounds and from different parts of Slovenia. I was getting to know Slovenia.

The fact that Slovenia had broken away from the 'communist Yugoslavia' only a couple of years earlier was quite evident and easily noticeable in the people, their general behaviour and in their mentality.

I was a guy with a somewhat shy kind of personality. Even though I was meeting people who were more open and more talkative than I was, there was still this constant feeling of pessimism or something in the 'background' and in their personality, which I simply could not, and did not want to, adapt to.

My first year in Slovenia went quite well. My studies progressed a little slowly, though. This was most likely also due to the language barrier. Perhaps the cultural background also played a small part. I was a typical youngster, studying, going around, meeting people, and basically living life.

My first year at university came to an end and it was time for my first summer holiday in Slovenia. My mother came to visit from South Africa. She came to spend some time with me and to organise and celebrate my 21'st birthday. That was the climax of my mother's visit to Slovenia. In Slovenia it's a person's 18th birthday which is celebrated 'big time'. But in South Africa it's the 21st birthday. I moved to Slovenia in between the two, so we decided to make a bit of a party for my 21'st birthday. I have relatives all around the country, but most of them live in the east. This is where I spent the majority of the summer break and where I also celebrated my birthday.

Well, that time came to an end and it was time for my mother to return to South Africa. Neither of us knew when we would see each other again, so for us to part was a little bit emotional. I saw her off and the next day I myself headed back 'home', towards Ljubljana. That, more or less, was the end of my summer break, before I was to start the next school year at the faculty.

Chapter three

I was heading back 'home', back to the relatives where I was living. The trip took quite some time even though it wasn't such a great distance. I had to take three different trains. But I didn't make it to my destination.

At first I didn't know what had happened to me or where I was. I woke up in the doctor's surgery, in a town close to where my relatives lived. I was informed that something had happened to me on the train, but they could not confirm exactly what. There were no witnesses, or, in other words, nobody who could describe what had actually happened to me.

The doctors weren't too concerned since they couldn't really confirm what it was and what had happened. Maybe I had just fainted or something. They obviously did not know the history of my health condition, and the accident or in other words the injuries I had obtained a year before. So, they just informed me to 'take it a bit easy' for a while and that was about it.

That is what I did. I still had time before the next school year started, so that is exactly how it was. There wasn't much to do, other than waiting for time to pass before the start of the next school year. My uncle associated it with having to part from my mother the day before. He added and expressed that I could be a little more independent since I was already over 20 years old.

A couple of days after the incident on the train, I was at home in the living room watching TV. All of a sudden, for no apparent reason, this awful drowsy feeling I had never experienced before came over me. I was alone, it frightened me and I panicked a bit too, "What was going on?" I got up to find somebody, to find help. I went into the hallway as my uncle was coming in the opposite direction. Feeling a bit anxious I reached out and said “Something’s wrong, help!”. That was it!

I woke up on the couch a while later with an awful headache and a not too pleasant feeling all over my body.

Now at least I had witnesses. Somebody who could describe to the doctors what they saw and what had happened to me. We returned to the doctor and my uncle described what he had seen.

They came to the conclusion that it must have been an epileptic seizure. “EPILEPTIC SEIZURE! WHAT IS THAT?”, was our initial reaction. This also placed the incident I had on the train a week before into an entirely new perspective. My doctor gave me a referral to go to the central hospital in Ljubljana to see a neurologist.

This was all happening just before the beginning of my second year at the faculty. I had been devoting quite a lot of attention to my studies, so going to the hospital for that check-up was more or less just something on the sidelines.

The neurologist confirmed that it was in fact epilepsy. A post-traumatic type of epilepsy, resulting from the injuries I had received a year before. This put quite a bit of emphasis on what had in fact happened on that mountainside and on the severity of the injuries I had obtained in the accident.

This placed my head injuries and the severity of those injuries in an entirely different perspective, compared to the time period directly after the accident, since I had recovered so well at that time.

I was given anti-epileptic medication which I had to take on a daily basis. I had no real problems taking it, and it quickly became a daily ritual. I had to take the medications twice a day, once in the morning and once in the evening. I also had regular check-ups by a neurologist who monitored my condition closely to see, amongst other things, how I was adapting to the medication and if there were any changes in the condition.

It went pretty well, because in the short period before I started taking these anti-epileptic medications, I was having about two seizures a week. But once I started taking the medication, the frequency of seizures dropped quite dramatically to about one seizure every two to three months.

All these new additions in life, having to take medication every day, and regular check-ups by a neurologist, came as I was in the second year of my studies. The second year was an exceptionally important one, because students had to decide and confirm which course and the direction they wanted to take to continue with their studies.

I decided on aeronautical engineering, a decision and desire I had made long before, even before I had completed high-school in South Africa.

Even though I was staring this awful medical condition, epilepsy, right in the face, I was still persistent with my desire to continue in the field of aeronautical engineering. Maybe I had not contemplated the full meaning and reality of the condition, and of what it meant for my life?

Well, life carried on quite normally. I eventually got used to the general flow of living. Going to the faculty every day, and having medical check-ups every now and then.

I eventually also started including a couple of new activities into my daily life. One such activity was that I became a member of the student organisation. Quite a large number of students study away from home, or, in other words, they come from all over the country and spend the week in the city, away from home and away from their parents.

The student organisation is involved with general life and activities for students, such as helping them find part-time jobs etc. Even though I became a member of the organisation, I still didn't get too involved with any additional activities.

I spent the majority of my free time at home. I always went home shortly after classes ended. I wasn't too enthusiastic about mingling with people. It was a common ritual for students to stop over at the pub for a quick drink and chat after classes. I just wasn't a very conversational or social type of guy. I generally got on the first train homeward bound. The most mingling I did was at weekends. I often went to the other side of the country to spend weekends with various relatives.

That's how life went on. Epilepsy and epileptic seizures were just part of my life. I was quite lucky because even though I did have the worst type of seizures, I was lucky that the frequency was reasonably low. The type of seizures I experience are referred to as 'grand mal' seizures, whereby I would fall down, lose consciousness and have minor trembling of my limbs.

It was quite fortunate that I had a reasonably low frequency of seizures, and a second stretch of luck was that I didn't ever have any while at university or practically anywhere away from home, where it could have caused panic amongst those who witnessed it. I hardly told anybody that I even had epilepsy. I always was a somewhat introvert and a fairly unsociable type of person in general.

Even though I was at home reasonably early every day, I used to spend the majority of the time in my room. Well, my studies took quite a lot of time. While at home I was comfortable spending time in my room doing all kinds of little activities along with my studies, not socialising much at all.

The weekends, which I so much enjoyed on the other side of the country visiting relatives, also became less. They weren't so enjoyable anymore. They had that, "it's not like it used to be" kind of feeling to them. I had a feeling that my relatives were to some extent trying to control my life, or at least wanting to make my decisions for me. As a result, I spent that much more time at home.

Even though I was at home more, I still didn't spend any more time with the relatives I was living with. I remember once when my uncle came into my room. He was concerned why I didn't want to spend time with them and asked why I spent so much time in my room, alone. We had a lengthy discussion, but I couldn't give him a concrete answer as to why I was like that.

Being so far away from home and far from my parents wasn't so easy, something my uncle also mentioned and, in doing so, showed his understanding. But then again, it wasn't so awfully difficult either. I couldn't quite explain it, I just enjoyed being by myself, in my room, doing 'my own' stuff.

I also spent quite a bit of time outdoors. I brought my bike with me from South Africa. I have always enjoyed cycling and it was something I wanted to carry on with in Slovenia. This only added to the dissatisfaction of my relatives. They didn't like it, how I was spending so little time with them. As if I had something against them, but I didn't. This is just the kind of person I am, something my relatives had a bit of a difficult time to accept.

The friction between me and my relatives only became worse. It wasn't as if I was arguing with them or anything like that. The atmosphere just wasn't what it could have been or what anybody would want it to be. But what could I do, I was just being the person I was.

Was this a sufficient reason to blame someone, because they are quieter, more personal and maybe a little more unsociable than you would like them to be?

The second year of my studies was coming to an end and summer was approaching. I was in fairly regular contact with my parents back in South Africa, as were my relatives. So, my parents were quite aware of the various goings on here in Slovenia and the general atmosphere in the relationship between me and my relatives.

This was the summer when my father was going to come and visit and it was going to be a summer with more great changes for me.

Chapter four

I was facing one of the greatest changes since moving to Slovenia. Almost as great as the decision I had made to leave home, my parents, my brothers, the life and surroundings I grew up in and was used to in South Africa and to move to Slovenia. I knew that I would face new challenges as a result, possibly greater than any I had ever faced so far. But it was a change I was willing to make and one I was actually looking forward to.

Since my father was here, we all together, my father, my relatives and I, sat down, talked and came to the conclusion that the best way to go from here would be for me to move out.

We then discussed how life was going to go from here. We had to resolve some concerns before I could finally move out.

The first and greatest challenge was to find a place, a room to rent, or somewhere where I could stay. Thankfully, it didn't take too long to find somewhere.

Life was about to go through some great changes.

I knew I would face new challenges as a result, but I wasn't really worried and was confident that I would be OK. What was most important to me was that I was finally independent. I could decide for myself what I wanted to do, where I wanted to go, everything.

I felt that I was opening up to people more than I had before. I became more conversational and sociable than I used to be. I also started enjoying social life more and got acquainted with the nightlife of Ljubljana.

The atmosphere at the faculty was changing too. Lectures were more relative to the direction of study I had selected. Classes were smaller, or in other words, the numbers of students in each class were now less than before. I got to know individual classmates better. Or maybe it was as a result of the changes I had made in my social life, that I was opening up more and thus got to know people better than I had previously. It was most probably a bit of both. But my circle of friends still remained reasonably small.

The independence I looked forward to so much also had its downsides and obligations. There was more I had to take care of. There was the washing, ironing, shopping and so forth.

There were so many new obligations, which went alongside taking care of my health. Since I had all these new issues and obligations I had to be more aware of, I actually became a great deal more focused on my health and my condition than I had been before. Well, I was alone now, so I kind of knew that I had to because there was nobody else there who I could lean on for support.

Even though there was so much going on in my life, my health condition and epilepsy had not changed dramatically. One change in my health though was my eyesight. I've never been sure if this had anything to do with the injury to my head, or the epilepsy. Or whether this was just a normal result of stressing my eyes too much because of my studies and other such activities.

Up until now the frequency of my epileptic seizures had not changed significantly. Maybe they had become a little less frequent, but not by much. I was lucky that the frequency of seizures was not too high, more or less three months between each. I just made sure that I was taking my medication. I still had reasonably regular check-ups with my neurologist, every couple of months. What I did notice, however, was that eating regularly, and eating enough, greatly influenced my wellbeing.

One advantage I have with my epilepsy is that I have these feelings before I have a seizure. They call it the aura effect. I found out that if I took quick enough action, the aura feeling would often ease off and go away. It also often happened that I had these aura feelings and they would go away without developing into a full epileptic seizure.

I was more comfortable with this independent way of life and even though there was so much more I had to do to take care of myself, the tempo of life was actually slowing down quite a bit. I eventually got used to the Slovene language and my studies were also progressing quite well.

The dropout rate at the faculty was quite high. About 60% of all the students who start off, normally drop out within the first two years. But I endured, even though progress was still slow and it was quite tough, I still pushed forward.

I also experienced my first epileptic seizure while at the faculty. As I mentioned previously, I had the advantage of the aura effect, which warned me that a seizure could be close. When I felt that the feeling was not going away, but getting stronger, I left the class to take a quick walk to see if that would maybe help. It unfortunately did progress into a full epileptic seizure and I fell in the hallway. Somebody called for help and the paramedics came. They took care of me and simply waited until I awoke and got back to my senses. They didn't see any valid reason to take me to the hospital.

One issue about this more independent way of life though was that I no longer had that place, that safety or comfort zone, where it would be more or less OK for me to have a seizure. I was aware that if it did happen, that it would most likely happen in the presence of strangers.

I also wasn't too comfortable or too open about talking to people about epilepsy. Almost nobody at university, or any of the other places I frequented, knew that I even had it. I was lucky that the experience I had while at the faculty went by with few witnesses.

I didn't talk that often with the landlady where I was living either, so even she didn't know that I had epilepsy. We normally always just greeted each other and had a little friendly chat here and there, every now and then, and that was about it.

Then one day it happened that I had a seizure while I was at home in my room. Even though I spent little time at home, it was obviously always destined to happen. A seizure was almost always followed by a period where I would become physically able, but I hadn't quite yet come to my senses. This also happened when I had the seizure at home. Following the seizure I went out of my room, downstairs to where the landlady lived. All I remembered was that all of a sudden, for no apparent reason, I was in her apartment. Only later did I realise and remember that I had had a seizure. Then all the unusual happenings of why I had gone down stairs all fell into place.

From here onwards the friendly relationship I had with my landlady went downhill. I realised and felt that since she learnt that I had epilepsy it seemed to mean to her that I was not the same person anymore.

Well, in this case it was understandable, since I was living there and, undoubtedly, it must have made her a bit uncomfortable and concerned. It's not as if it got really unpleasant or anything. I just realised that it was not quite the same as it was before she knew I had epilepsy.

It was instances like the one at 'home' with the landlady, that only made it more uncomfortable and more difficult for me to talk about epilepsy.

But on the other hand, there were those experiences which had quite positive results. As I mentioned previously, classes at the faculty were getting smaller and I was getting to know individual classmates better. I had a circle of friends who I knew I could trust and with whom I had a really good friendship with. These were the kind of people who I did tell that I had epilepsy, because I felt comfortable enough to be able to freely talk with them about my condition.

One day the most undesirable happened. The one thing I believe the majority of people with epilepsy fear or dislike the most. We were walking outside in the city with my friends, when I had a seizure. Since I was with these friends who knew I had epilepsy, they weren't too shocked when it happened and they also knew how to react and what to do to help me.

The incident with my friends clearly showed me the benefits of acquainting people about my condition. I think I became more open to the fact that I had epilepsy and also more open to sharing the fact with others.

As life went on and became more settled, I started including more social activities. One of these was that I helped out at a church. I was leading one of four groups of an English conversational class which they organized. This meant that I was mingling more with strangers. Thus, I also became more comfortable with the reality of having epilepsy and the possibility of me having a seizure amongst strangers.

Chapter five

It was Tuesday evening. Another day of English conversational classes. But today, 14th of February 1998, was also Valentine's Day. So, we used Valentine's Day as the main topic of conversation. Towards the end of classes all the groups came together in the kitchen to bake cookies. The atmosphere was good and very sociable. I met all the students, including those from other groups. I was much more comfortable and more talkative when using the English language, so I was a lot more sociable than normal.

One of the students, a keen traveller who wanted to retain her knowledge of the English language, spoke fluent English and was especially friendly. She even offered to drive me home after class. The next Tuesday this student moved to my group and after class we went out for a short walk. That is when it all started. I was eventually getting to know somebody, Breda, her nickname was 'Bina', the name her niece and nephews gave her.

We were in regular contact with each other, and not only for English conversational classes. We were meeting more and more often. Mostly taking walks through Ljubljana, chatting and getting to know each other. Reasonably quickly it went that far that we started holding hands. Something was blossoming here.

Then one day as we were walking, I stopped and turned to her. I looked her in the eyes, "There's something I've got to tell you, something you don't know", I said. She anxiously waited as I continued. "I have epilepsy", I said.

I was at that point again, where I had been so many times before. At that point when people find out you have epilepsy, then it changes everything, when, all of a sudden, you're not the same person you were before. But this time it turned out differently. She accepted me!

Our relationship carried on from there, as if I hadn't even told her. That was also her reaction. She didn't really mind and it didn't really bother her that I had epilepsy. I was still a little worried though, at what her reaction would be if, or when, she would actually witnesses a seizure.

Our relationship grew. We spent more and more time together and we got to know each other better and better.

I constantly monitored my wellbeing and the frequency of my epileptic seizures. Sometimes I would have good periods, when I would feel pretty good with few auras and when the frequency of seizures would drop. And then I would have bad periods when I would have constant auras, sometimes several in a single day and also the frequency of seizures would be higher. But then again, the frequency of seizures didn't really fluctuate so much.

It was during this period, when I was getting to know Bina, that the frequency of my seizures actually dropped. Was the way I was feeling in general; excited with love blossoming, in a good mood etc., actually having an effect on the epilepsy? Or was it just a coincidence? There was this fluctuation of the frequency of seizures and how I was feeling. But I didn't really pay much attention to finding out why this may have been.

Life progressed at a steadier rate now. Our relationship blossomed and we grew closer to each other. My studies also progressed, and my social life was also coming along well. After some time, Bina and I decided that I would move in with her. Since I was living alone, renting a room, the decision to move was not a hard one to make.

It was now the third time in six years that I had moved. Each time, it was not only a change of location, but also a complete change of atmosphere. I once again had that place I could comfortably call 'home'.

It was about a year-and-a-half after I moved in with Bina, that we got married.

We had a few concerns about having children. Even though I was not the one who would conceive, we still pondered the possibility of epilepsy being inherited. I had heard about children inheriting epilepsy. Seriously thinking about becoming parents, we were obviously worried. My neurologist was kind enough to talk to both of us about our concerns. He comforted us that in my case it would not happen, since I was suffering from post-traumatic epilepsy. That was a great relief for both of us and we could start creating our own family, with one less worry on our minds.

In September 2000 our daughter was born. Bina had gone into the maternity unit a couple of days before, because of some minor concerns. They said they would call me to come in when Bina went into labour. The birth took quite some time. It was about 15 hours after they called me to come to the maternity unit until Sarah was eventually born.

It was these important events, such as our wedding and again when Sarah was born, which had this bit of fear and concern always hanging over them. "Will I make it through this without having a seizure", or, "I hope I'll be OK ...". It's not as if I would over-exaggerate about it, but there was still this constant concern in the back of my mind, reminding me. But when the event or whatever would start and my mind and thoughts were kept busy, I would forget about the epilepsy altogether.

It was during instances when that aura feeling would come along, while I was out somewhere, in the presence of strangers or when I was in the presence of a larger group of people. These were the instances that I hated the most. Those were quite unpleasant feelings, knowing and regularly being reminded that 'the worst' could happen.

Then, one day when we were out in public, I had a seizure. Bina had got tickets to watch a well-known comedian. So, it was obviously an opportunity not to be missed. This was the worst place to have a seizure, where it could interrupt the show and for absolutely everyone present, which I obviously would not want at all. But what was unique about this comic was that he is also a doctor, who turned comedian. So, when he noticed that there was something wrong, he automatically stopped the show to come to my assistance. A very embarrassing moment, but Bina said that he took really good control of the situation and ensured that the show still carried on and that, in the end, it didn't turn out too badly. Something I think anybody with epilepsy would never want to happen, but which turned out better than I thought it would.

Similar concerns, such as, "I hope I'll be OK", would also arise when we, or even more when I alone, would go on a trip. But most of the time we would only remember this and make comments about it after everything was over. We would comment on how fortunate it was that all went well and that I didn't have any problems. Obviously, the fact that I had such a low frequency of seizures, meant that I could do so much more, and as time went on that concern, "What if I have any problems?", became less and less. It was clear that we sometimes over-exaggerated with our worries and concerns.

Sarah brought some great and beautiful things into our lives and into our home, such as the blessings and also challenges of parenthood. At first I didn't have much to do since newborn babies are still so fragile and so dependent on their mothers. But slowly, as time went on, my role and obligations as a father came into action and I slowly but surely became more involved in being with, and taking care, of Sarah.

Bina's year of maternity leave soon ended, and she had to return to work. Since I had not yet completed my studies, I was in a period of doing my studies and odd jobs here and there. I even had a couple of jobs I did from home. It was therefore easy for me to adapt my schedule and any commitments accordingly.

I also had the responsibility of taking care of Sarah while Bina was at work. At first I was hardly ever alone with Sarah, so if a seizure did come on, I always had somebody close by. Even if it meant that I was outside and the other people were strangers, I was careful to ensure I was never entirely alone with Sarah, just in case I did unfortunately have a seizure when I was with her.

There was only one such instance when I was taking care of Sarah while Bina was at work, that I had a seizure. I was at home. As I felt the aura getting stronger, I got Sarah and took her into the next room to my mother-in-law. Everything turned out okay in the end. I did have a seizure, but Sarah was alright.

It was about a year after Bina returned to work that Sarah started going to kindergarten. Luckily there had only been this one single event which reminded us of the risks and possible dangers which were constantly present in everything I was doing. But these were risks I was willing to take. Since the frequency of seizures was so low, and even though I had had this one incident which was a constant reminder of the risks, I started spending more and more time with Sarah. We spent a great deal of time outside, going to the park, to the shops and to the city to wait for Bina as she finished work.

As time went on I started getting ever more confident in spending more and more time with Sarah, even if we were alone. Family life was progressing quite prosperously.

Chapter six

It was in this period not long after moving in with Bina and when Sarah was born, that the rest of my family started moving over from South Africa.

My brother was the first to move. He moved to Slovenia in 1997, settled in quite quickly, found a job and a place to live. A few years later my mother moved over too. We had a yacht in South Africa so my father remained there to finalise moving out of the country and to prepare his journey to Slovenia by yacht. My mother was not too keen to come all the way up the Atlantic and through the Mediterranean by yacht, so she moved over earlier.

We did not live together. My brother had his apartment in a neighbouring city, not far away. My mother and brother lived together for some time. We saw each other quite often and spent quite a lot of time together, especially with my mother who really quickly got acquainted with Bina and Sarah.

My father eventually did make the epic journey and arrived in Slovenia just a couple of months before the 10th anniversary of my epic move here.

My family knew that I had epilepsy, but none of them have ever witnessed me having a seizure. At first I spoke little about it, so they did not know the full reality of the condition. My mother was most curious about my condition and about epilepsy in general and had many questions about my wellbeing. Of course, it was her mother's instinct, and she obviously wanted to know what was going on with her son. But she wasn't too keen on the idea of me having a seizure in front of her. Understandingly, she never wanted to see it. Fortunately, we didn't live together so the chance of that happening was slim.

My parents settled in quite quickly. They moved into the house where my father was born and spent his childhood. It was quite a distance away, but we still saw each other fairly often. My father found a job where he could make good use of the experience and knowledge he had gained during his working career in South Africa, so we saw a little less of each other. I was in regular contact with my mother and started to share more about epilepsy and my condition with her, especially when my interest started to grow, and I had more I could tell her about it. I had more theories and medical facts, I could share with her. Through this I believe I also showed that I was quite comfortable living with it and that I had accepted that I was suffering from the condition.

It was somewhat interesting and I was actually quite surprised at the different reactions of my parents, reactions I would never have predicted. Firstly I felt right away how my father fell directly into the taboo of what a devastating medical abnormality epilepsy is, and that whatever is wrong with me for certainly cannot be epilepsy, trying to constantly push the reality of the situation aside. He would often continue with that what I am suffering from is “not epilepsy.” I was surprised that, even as the years went on, his interpretation or comments didn’t change much.

My mother, on the other hand was different and her reaction was most surprising and unexpected. She actually was a little interested in epilepsy and wanted to know what it meant and what it was like to have seizure. Though, she did not like to talk about it too much and she declared that she would never like to see me having a seizure. It was understandable that she never wanted to see a seizure. As the years went by her perspective changed quite a great deal. It was true that I spoke more with her about the condition and about my wellbeing. Maybe it was because of this, that she changed her perspective. I was surprised when she once said, "Maybe it would be better for me to see you having a seizure". She continued that she would then get a real perspective of what it really is like, that it may not be as bad as she was always thinks it is.

I think it was a very wise and a good and understanding reaction I got from my mother, I must say. Totally contrary to the taboo my father and many people create of how much of a devastating abnormality epilepsy is.

Chapter seven

And, as they always say, “Life carries on”. Yes, it did, and I and my family went with it. I found a permanent job and was able to more comfortably support myself and my family. It did however take quite some time, before I eventually found a permanent and stable job though. It might have been a period that was packed with various concerns and challenges, but it was also a period which brought much learning and experience in various areas.

In that time, I worked in a number of different fields, for example when I was still busy with my studies I worked for a garden service. It was nice working there. It is an organisation, which covers all kinds of garden work and work with plants; general gardening, gardens in front of offices and even taking care of plants for a number of town councils. Whilst there, I made friends with people I am still in contact with today, and I gained some valuable experience in gardening; working with plants and with garden tools.

Then there were also a couple of odd building and renovation jobs that I helped out with and where I again gained valuable knowledge and experience, which would come in handy later in life.

I also realised that when I was in almost constant motion, or, in other words, when I was physically active, I never had any problems or even any unpleasant feelings i.e. that aura feeling, related to the epilepsy.

It took some time for me to find a permanent job. This only meant that I had that much more appreciation and gratitude when I did eventually find one. Additionally, it was the kind of work I really enjoyed doing - designing and drawing equipment - ‘technical drawing’. This was really valuable and important to me, to be able to do the kind of work I enjoyed.

I was aware that my epilepsy was a serious matter when it came to my occupation. I had read quite a bit about it, about the various concerns and even more; The experiences people had when it came to putting the two together, epilepsy and their occupation. There had only been one single experience that I had during those part time jobs I did in the past. Not that I had a seizure, but simply because I told the people there that I had epilepsy. You know how it goes from there, all of a sudden you become a different person.

It was from what I found out and from what I myself experienced, that I became a bit more cautious. I decided not to tell anybody at work that I had epilepsy. It was obviously a bit of a gamble, but I took a risk and hoped that I would not have a seizure too soon, before they got to know me well enough. I have this philosophy, 'Let them get to know you, to see what you are really capable of and then later, when appropriate, let them know that you have epilepsy'.

In Slovenia it is normal to have a trial-period before a company permanently employs you. In most cases it lasts up to about half a year. "If only I could get through this stage, then when the atmosphere and the ideal opportunity would arise, I could let them know I have epilepsy", was the way I thought I'd do it. Who knows, maybe this is not quite the correct approach to take, maybe I would never find that 'ideal moment' to let the people know. Even if that 'ideal moment' did come along, would I take full advantage of it? An issue full of questions. But this is how I did it.

It is a lot easier to get to know people well enough and for them to get to know you before you tell them something like this. There were one or two colleagues who I felt I could trust and with whom I felt comfortable enough talking about my condition. I liked the attitude of one of them, who said something like, "Well, what can you do? You've just got to accept it and make the best of life and move forward". A very true and logical way of looking at any such situation.

Then, obviously, it did happen, the thing I had feared the most. I still remember the day very well. The day at work when that unwelcome and unpleasant aura feeling came along. The aura became stronger and didn't seem to go away. I knew that this was not going to be good, so I got up to get some water to drink and a breath of fresh air, but it was too late. I had barely left our section and gone into the main hallway before I fell and had a seizure.

It happened right next to the director's office. I also hurt myself a little in the fall. It obviously caused a bit of a panic among pretty much everybody in the building, since practically nobody knew about my condition. But in the end I felt that I had succeeded. I had managed to show my employer and all the others of what I am capable and who I really am, that I take my obligations in the workplace seriously. This kind of overpowered the reality and any such negative impacts of me having epilepsy.

I was already back at work the next day. In the days that followed I had a talk with my supervisor, and also with the director. I explained to them why I chose not to tell them about my epilepsy from the start, as I logically should have. I described some of the experiences I had had in the past, of the kind of reactions I had received when I did tell people. I also chatted quite a bit with the rest of my colleagues who I was, and still am, in closer contact with. There are quite a number of us in the section where I work, so we have had quite a lot of discussions about epilepsy and the various experiences I had in the past. I got quite a positive reaction from practically all of the people in the company who just accepted that I suffer from the condition. For the majority of people, I was pretty much the same person I was the day before, capable of all my obligations in the workplace, which was most important.

I realised that the people at work did not put as much emphasis on the fact that I had epilepsy, as some other people had done in the past. They accepted me as the person I am, capable of carrying out my obligations and taking my job seriously.

That obviously wasn't the only time I have ever had a seizure at work, and I knew and expected that it wouldn't be the last time either. It was also fortunate that the people in the organisation, especially the director, are very logical, understanding and know that we are all human beings.

There was one experience though which I believe did bring some changes in the way my closer colleagues looked at the fact that I was a person with epilepsy. We had a ritual in our section that at the end of each year, before the Christmas and New Year break, we would go out for a fun and social afternoon together. Most of the time we would go bowling, or play pool. It was one of these days, when we had all gone out together, first for a drink, then on to the pool-hall, It was while playing pool that I had a seizure.

These were the experiences I dreaded the most. When the intention was to have fun or a good time with people, and then for me to have a seizure, which then most definitely ruins the social atmosphere. Not only for me, but what bothered me more, was that it would most definitely ruin, or at least alter, the atmosphere for everybody else present.

Having a permanent job obviously brought changes into my life in general, one of which was the great relief and improved order to the general tempo of life. Not only could I take better care of all those important obligations in life, taking care of my family, finances, etc, but it actually gave me a better feeling of freedom. Since some of those major concerns were now taken care of, I actually found more opportunity for extra casual and social activities and I could even put more emphasis on those activities that I wanted to spend more time on in my spare time.

It is interesting how, even though a greater part of the day was now being taken up, I actually started finding new activities. The atmosphere and feelings of all other activities had also changed. Even though I now had even less time for my casual activities, I felt that I could enjoy them better. Having a permanent job means a lot more than just being able to take care of those important obligations in life.

Chapter eight

One of those extra activities that I was going to start spending more time on, was my interest in epilepsy. With time, I came to realise that there was a lot more to the condition than just taking your medication and regularly visiting a neurologist, listening and doing only what they might recommend.

Once while chatting with my mother on the telephone, she mentioned something she had heard on the radio. It was about the advantages of fish oil, or omega-3 oil as it is also called, for people with epilepsy. I hadn't heard of this before, so I went onto the internet to see if I could find out more. I found quite a lot of interesting facts and explanations substantiating the benefits and effects of omega-3 oil for those suffering from epilepsy and for brain health in general, so I decided to try it out.

In addition, I found more and more interesting articles about the effects of nutrition on epilepsy. I always knew and had a strong feeling that nutrition was important, both for my wellbeing in general and to be able to cope a little more easily with the condition. But I was not quite sure of any specific details.

Other realisations were some general observations that Bina and I were making about my condition and daily life in general. Since we were living together and spending so much more time together, it was easier for both of us to notice how, and which issues influenced and effected my wellbeing more than others. It was more in the sense of what to avoid, or rather, which situations or surroundings would have a greater effect on my wellbeing. One of those was the importance of fresh air.

Progress was slow but sure. I started realising that much of what I actually did myself, greatly influenced my wellbeing.

I was quite content with life and with what I had achieved so far. I had found true love and started creating my own family. I had found a job doing something that I enjoyed, which brought me great satisfaction in life, while, at the same time, I was able to take care of those many obligations of being a father and husband.

It was an ideal time and opportunity for our family to 'expand', so that is exactly what we did. We decided to have a second child. This time, it took quite a bit longer than we had expected for Bina to conceive. But we were successful and our second child was "on its way". It might have taken quite some time, but Sarah now had a brother, Timmy.

But that was not the end of the 'expansion', because we soon realised that it would be good to find a new home. The apartment we were living in was becoming too small.

It didn't take long for us to find a house. It was a house that entirely fulfilled our expectations and one which matched our pockets, or rather, our financial capabilities.

It was a reasonably old house that had been empty for some time. It was going to need quite a lot of renovation and modification. But I saw that as a positive, because it meant that I could do all the renovations and modifications according to how and to what we wanted. To suit our taste and desires. I knew this was going to be something I was going to enjoy doing. This was where all that experience I had gained in the past, from all those part-time jobs I had done, was going to come in handy. I spent a great deal of time in the house, involved in all kinds of building work and alterations, before we eventually moved in. This meant that I was oftentimes away from Bina and the children, but they came to the house almost every day to see what 'daddy' was doing. I liked including the children in any way I could in the work I was doing in and around the house.

This was all happening when Timmy was about two years old, cautiously toddling around, curiously exploring the world around him. I initially took care of all the larger projects which needed to be done, so that we could at least move into the house.

Even when we did move in, the house would still require a great deal of work, but we could at least comfortably live there.

Another 'move' that had to be arranged was that Sarah was going to have to change schools. She was only in the first grade when we moved. So now she was going to have to do it all over again. A new school, new surroundings, finding new friends, everything. But she 'fell right in', and found new friends. And the school also 'found her'.

Somebody in the school noticed her athletic capabilities and right away recommended that she try out for the triathlon team. The town has a very competitive triathlon team, and she once again Sarah 'fell straight in'. Whoever noticed this in her, obviously knew what they were looking at. It was excellent because these were the kind of sports I also took part in and enjoyed as a youngster, and had carried on with at an amateur level.

As parents, Bina and I also got quite involved with the club in various triathlon events. I really enjoyed it, firstly supporting Sarah in her activities and then also getting involved in the community. We met a lot of other families who also had children competing and were also involved in the club, or they themselves competed in triathlons.

I strongly believe that my general way of thinking, and also the way I faced all that life brought, played an important role in me being able to get so far, despite the additional challenges of suffering from epilepsy. Even without it, life would have been challenging enough. But I still managed to get 'far', move forward and live a pretty normal and decent life. It was this inner optimism and confidence I felt deep inside which helped me achieve a great deal.

Interestingly, I didn't have a strong sense of self-worth, whenever I thought 'directly' about myself or 'if I looked at myself in the mirror'.

When I got into a project, whether at home while working on the house, at work, or anywhere, I would put a great deal of effort into it. The level of endurance I had to strive and finish anything I tackled helped me the most. It was this level of endurance which has helped me accept and overcome so many of the challenges I have faced since arriving in Slovenia. Not only the challenges I faced because of epilepsy, but rather those kinds of challenges a person normally faces in life.

Chapter nine

It had become quite a busy period, as I had all kinds of renovation and building projects going on at home. But I also made time for the family, for Timmy and for Sarah.

I became a member of the parent-teacher association at Sarah's school. I liked how they involved parents in the school and in the lives of the children. The parents were called together, obviously those who volunteered, to decorate the school. It was getting close to the festive season so the parents and children decorated the hallways.

An even greater event was the school bazaar. The pupils would create all kinds of items they would then sell. The school also pitched in and bought a variety of items that the pupils could then sell at the bazaar. It was quite a big event which stretched over a couple of days.

On one of the days, Sarah and I decided to see what was going on at the school, and we spent quite a long time there. Then I started getting those minor aura feelings, so I decided that we had had enough and it would be good to get out and go home.

But it was too late. I had barely made it out of the school building when I had a seizure. I fell and hit my head on a concrete ventilation duct. Bystanders reacted quickly and somebody called for an ambulance and I was rushed off to hospital.

Because I had had a seizure, I obviously didn't have any recollection of what had happened to me. I don’t know if I woke up in the ambulance. I can only vaguely remember being in hospital after waking up more or less a week after the incident.

Looking back at the whole incident, I don't even remember how long I was in hospital or even when I came home. I can still remember the first time I was in hospital, after I had the accident back in 1994. But this time, more than ten years later, nothing. The first moments I do remember was when I was at home, slowly recovering, more than a month after the incident by the school. So in other words, more than a month of my life was just gone, a 'black hole'. But this was just the beginning, just a fraction of what I was about to experience.

My recovery at home went really slowly. I remember being up in my room, spending a lot of time in bed resting. At first I got up for short periods, just to change location and to walk around a little in the house. Recovery was really slow.

One of the events which melted itself deep into my soul, one I still remember so clearly, was being in the room upstairs, lying down and having my four-year-old son there with me. He eventually became more comfortable around me. He was being the excited four-year-old that he was, so full of energy and life. Having my own son there, his presence and excitement, should have been something pleasant, but inside me I didn’t feel anything, no feelings, nothing! But that wasn't all. That was only the start, the first incident which made such an impression. An impression I would never forget. It didn't matter who I was with, whether it with Bina, Sarah or Timmy, or even my mother, who was often around after this incident, I felt nothing. But this was only the beginning of what I was going to experience.

I was about to experience a side of epilepsy that I had only read and heard about, but had never paid much attention to.

My physical recovery went quite steadily at first, but there was at least some progress. I started becoming more mobile, more able and more independent.

But psychologically, I felt such little progress, if any at all. I didn't realise the extent or the condition of my psyche, I just knew that things were not right. This was so different compared to physical injuries, which almost always recover in time. I had regular check-ups by a neurologist and, for the first time ever, also visits to a psychiatrist.

I also had a loss of short-term memory. On the one hand, this short-term memory loss, though unpleasant, also had its interesting sides, as I was putting more emphasis and effort into trying to remember things. I realised that I could easily remember quite irrelevant details of events which may have happened years before. I could remember them so well and in such detail as if they had happened more recently. But more recent events were at times a lot harder to remember than the older ones. It was unbelievable.

Another specific and greater challenge was remembering names. Whether it was the names of people, places, whatever, it didn't matter. I simply had great difficulty in remembering names.

I was going to be at home for quite some time before I would be able to go back to work, or before life would, at least a little, return back to that normal and active tempo I was so used to. Even though my physical recovery was going quite well and progress was becoming greater and greater as time went on, I still took it easy. For some time, the greatest activity for me would be when I went by train to the city for one of the various medical check-ups I had to have.

I was really proud of myself when I eventually independently walked the whole distance from the train station to the rehabilitation centre where I had the check-ups. Even though it was less than two kilometres, I was still proud of being able to do it independently.

Since there had been such good progress with my physical capabilities, I started taking more and more notice of that one part of my life which was not progressing at all, and which was becoming so much more obvious. One really important and vital part of almost any physical activity is that feeling of satisfaction or success of what you have done. This was so missing.

I knew that these missing feelings were somehow associated to those feelings, or I should rather say, “lack of feelings”, that I had experienced right at the beginning, when I had Timmy in my room, and then later, those 'missing feelings' for everybody around me.

All those ’missing feelings’ had common similarities, and were missing almost everywhere in what life had for me. As I was becoming physically ever more and more mobile and independent, travelling around more and being active and independent in all kinds of activities around the house and elsewhere, this emptiness was becoming greater and greater and I started to increasingly notice it. To cut it short, a great deal of my psyche had simply gone. What I missed most were the feelings I had as a father for my children, and those that I had had as a husband to Bina.

This lack of feelings bothered me tremendously. I was searching in all kinds of ways to try and find them and get them back. As time went on, and as I was becoming increasingly physically active and independent, those missing pieces started bothering me more and more.

With time, I realised that through physical activity and keeping myself busy in any kind of way, I could at least keep my mind busy, thus not putting so much emphasis and thoughts on these missing feelings. You could say I was kind of avoiding them.

With time and through great effort, those feelings would eventually start coming back. But not all of them and those that did start coming back, would at first, only came back in small pieces.

Firstly, the feelings I had for my children. I don't know if it was because I was putting so much emphasis and effort into 'finding' those feelings again, but the love, respect and gratitude I had for my children was becoming so acute and amazing. Though it was obviously going to take quite some time for all this to happen, at least I could feel some real progress being made here too.

Unfortunately, this wasn't the case for all the feelings I was so dearly searching for. The feelings I had for Bina were somewhat different. I couldn't quite understand it, but the feelings for my wife, which I too so dearly missed, just didn't budge and simply weren't there.

Slowly I also started to realise the value of the efforts I was putting into my recovery. I started putting a great amount of effort and emphasis on recovering and was certainly able to feel the results of those efforts.

Thinking back on the whole experience, I am so grateful that my mind and my psyche were at least sufficient enough for me to realise that there was something wrong, that there was something missing. Because without that, I wouldn't have had the desire to get it back and I certainly wouldn't have put any effort into it. The essays and various information I found on the internet were of great help. Some of them described so well what I was feeling and experiencing. This helped me more easily understand what I was feeling and going through and that I wasn't alone with what I was experiencing.

Eventually, the medical check-ups became less frequent, and I felt I could maybe even return to work. I spoke to my neurologist and returned to work long before the doctors predicted I would be able to. I described the kind of work I do and that I felt confident that I was capable of returning to work.

At first I started working for only four hours, but it wasn't long before I started working for the full eight hours. Going back to work wasn't easy, and, although I knew it was going to be challenging, in the end it was a lot more so than I had imagined it would be. Firstly, the problems I had with memory loss caused quite a few challenges. But what caused even greater challenges was the difficulties I had in remembering names. The full extent of the memory loss and all the other similar challenges I had, were only now becoming evident.

I still recall so clearly how I was trying to remember the names of my co-workers, I was surprised that three of them had the same surname. With a little pondering I remembered, "Oh of-course, how stupid of me, they're brothers and the one downstairs is their father". This was a clear indication of the extent of the memory loss I had experienced.

Since my work involves projects for various organisations and companies, the challenges of trying to remember and correctly place the names of these organisations caused quite a few difficulties. And there were going to be quite a number of challenges ahead in order that I would be able to successfully and independently do some of the tasks I had previously. I never expressed this to anybody, about this defect in my mind. I felt that I was still managing quite alright.

Since my mind, my thoughts and my feelings still had so much missing, other thoughts and feelings started taking their place. And obviously, when you are missing feelings of love and when your body, your mind and practically everything has these missing feelings, I think I don't need to explain what replaces them. Loneliness! Even though I always had Bina, the kids and other people physically close by, it didn't make much difference. There was this great gap of emptiness.

I preferred it when I at least had a task or something else to do to keep me and my mind busy. I still clearly remember when I started laying the driveway. This was going to be the first greater task or project that I was going to get into after the incident which had placed me in hospital. Maybe I was a bit selfish by acting and thinking in this kind of way. To be working, partially so that I could be alone, avoiding and being 'apart' from people and my family. Away and avoiding all those issues which were so lacking in life and which were bothering me so much. This obviously wasn't the right thing to do, or what anybody in their right mind would do. But what else could I do? This was one way, one 'place' where I found some comfort, some respite from all the troubles I was going through.

This didn't in any way mean that I stopped putting effort into finding my feelings and getting them back.

But these missing feelings didn't end only with feelings for my family. Those were just the feelings I noticed at first and those that were 'right at the top' of all of it, of all that was missing.

Because of everything that was going on, I didn't have much of a desire to mingle with people in general either. As a result of the memory loss, it would often happen that I would 'run into' people who would greet me, but I couldn't quite remember them, or from where and why I knew them. I simply greeted them back. This happened mostly in town because I would run into people, either from the triathlon club or other parents from Sarah's school.

Life was progressing, piece-by-piece, one step at a time. Slowly returning to what I was more or less used to, but there were these additional challenges and feelings I was facing in regard to my psyche.

There were so many portions of life that were progressing and returning to the norm that I was more or less familiar with: I was back at work and doing all kinds of tasks and work around the house etc. But this just served to make those parts which were still missing so much more evident. What eventually started becoming more present in my mind were thoughts of death and even suicide. Not that they were too frequent, but with time they became quite intense. I would often remember and think about a few accidents I had witnessed in my life, about those people who had lost their lives practically in front of me.

I must say, that even though I had so many challenges with my psychological wellbeing amongst others, I didn't ever feel that I had become really depressed or anything. I was quite content with life and the progress I was making. But the thoughts of suicide were still present. They were more like an unwanted presence in my mind and my thoughts. Something of an unwanted guest who sometimes simply just didn't want to leave. Thoughts of losing my life, whether through an accident or in any other way, plagued my mind quite a lot.

Apart from these thoughts of suicide and dying, I felt that I was making quite decent progress, that life in all aspects was slowly but surely returning to what it had been like before.

It was some time towards the end of 2009 when I heard and started taking notice of Facebook. At first I wasn't too interested because there were also quite a number of criticisms about it. It wasn't until I received an e-mail from an old school friend in South Africa, who recommended I get on Facebook so that we could get in contact. Only then did I start to take more notice of its advantages, especially for me. I quickly started getting in contact with quite a number of old school friends.

At the same time my relationship and the feelings I had for Sarah and Timmy were constantly developing and growing into something really special. I started spending more and more time with them. I found all kinds of ways to involve them in tasks around the house. But it didn't end there. With time this appreciation, respect and, you could say, love only increased even more and with time I had a special respect for children in general.

What did suffer, though, was my relationship with Bina. It was entirely lacking any sexual attraction or desire. This was one issue that was totally and utterly dormant in me. It also took quite a long time before I even realised that it was missing, because I didn't really miss it or even think about it. Thus, I was obviously not putting any emphasis on it or giving the matter any attention as I was doing with all those other feelings which I did realise were missing.

Another thing that was still lacking, and at which I was making very little progress, was the desire to mingle. I wasn't too enthusiastic, if at all. Whenever anyone came to visit, I mostly just avoided them and always had something to do around the house. And often, when the rest of the family went out somewhere, I stayed at home. OK, in some respects this was understandable since there was always some kind of work going on around the house. But then again, maybe I could have gone out a bit more than I actually did. Believe me, I remember what I was thinking and what I was going through. It wasn't as simple as just 'saying', "OK! Today we'll go ...". I would have very much liked it to have been that simple, but it wasn't. I don't know and cannot explain why.

Over time, I started reading more and acquainting myself more about epilepsy, especially about the psychological issues related to the condition. Even though there was some progress in my psyche, I was aware that there was still a great deal missing. I read about an issue referred to as the "psychosocial disorder", and started reading quite a bit about what this 'disorder' involves, what effect it has on people, and also how people react to it.

I found out quite a lot regarding the statistics of suicide amongst people suffering from epilepsy and also personal accounts of what others had experienced. I realised that the things going on in my mind weren't just coincidental but in fact were quite common. I found a number of articles which made quite an impression on me, and which so closely described what I was experiencing. I also read about where this had led other people and began to find out where this could lead me.

There were a couple of incidences that I will never forget. Times when I would think how quickly this could all be over. Just one step or one single action was all that was needed. It was horrible! It was in the middle of one such incident, when I was on my way somewhere and was taking the final steps onto the platform at the railway station, when those stupid uninvited thoughts of suicide again flooded my mind. But this time the experience made such an impression on me that I finally decided, **"This is definitely not the way I want to go anymore!!"**

It was quite understandable that this came to mind as I was on the platform at the railway station, since I had seen a number of accidents on railway platforms in the past, and these had always remained on the edges of my mind.

Since I travelled by trains quite frequently, it wasn't surprising that I witnessed accidents there. It was the memories of these accidents that now made me even change the way I waited and got onto the train. I waited somewhat away from the platform until the train arrived, and then went onto the platform and onto the train after it had arrived. This was another clear indication of how much these thoughts that were constantly plaguing my mind really bothered me. So much so that I even changed my typical daily habits and routine.

It was these events, all the reading and research I was doing about my condition, and obviously what I was going through, which influenced me, the way I was thinking, and ultimately the effort I was putting into being positive and optimistic.

What bothered me though was my sociability. I was putting a great effort into being more sociable and positively minded. But the two together - being more sociable and at the same time positively minded - were actually proving quite difficult. Especially here in Slovenia, where the two rarely go hand-in-hand, because when people get together for a chat, even if it's about the weather, the discussions generally always involve some pessimistic content, or are simply pessimistically orientated. This was one of the characteristics that I noticed in Slovenian people, quite soon after arriving. It was a characteristic I simply couldn't, and did not want to, associate myself with.

I decided that these factors were going to become the backbone of the person I would like to become, i.e. being positive and optimistic and also more sociable. The first of these was not going to be so difficult, since I was previously more or less positively minded, but being sociable was going to be a greater challenge, one which I would have to put a great amount of effort into.

But even being more positively minded was going to have its challenges. It was those undesirable and irregular pessimistic thoughts that would only add to the challenge. Whenever any of those stupid irritating thoughts about death, or whatever, came into my mind, I always tried replacing them by thinking about something else, anything else.

The combination of the special feelings I had for Sarah and Timmy, together with the fact that I was trying to be more sociable, was starting to become interesting. It was because of these special feelings I had for my own, and for children in general, that I started to notice young children more and also came into contact with some families with whom I would regularly cross paths in town.

Since children had a special place in my heart and my thoughts, I started taking more notice of the role of mothers and had added feelings of respect towards them. The mother of every child is the one who conceives, goes through some great changes and challenges as she carries her child for nine months before she goes through that, though painful, special moment of giving birth. And since I didn't feel as much sexual attraction towards women, these feelings of respect absolutely dominated my mind and became something really special to me. Whenever I saw a pregnant lady, I often had these thoughts, like a little prayer for her, wishing her well and good health. Maybe a little unusual and somewhat difficult to explain.

I eventually started becoming more sociable too. But I felt that I was being more sociable with strangers, rather than being in the company of people I knew well. Whenever I went anywhere where I would be in the presence of people I knew well, a picnic or similar, I so often just couldn't get into or join in on conversations. I don’t know why this was, but it often bothered me. It was common for me to say to myself,

"Oh man! Can't you be a bit more sociable ...". I often felt as if I didn't fit in.

I sometimes simply avoided such events that would mean being together with people, like picnics, parties and visits. My family often went out without me, while I did all kinds of tasks around the house.

One other portion of my social life which was going to become special, was the contact I had with people via Facebook, even though I wasn't such a fan of it at first. But what was special was that I started getting in contact with old school friends from South Africa. There were certain Facebook friends whose friendship meant so much to me that it was even worth spending the money to make some short international calls just to say "Hi!".

But even with all the social progress I was making, there was still this one very important portion which was practically going nowhere. My relationship with Bina. It's not as if we would get into arguments or anything like that. But there was that one great portion still missing. Was this somehow associated with my lack of sexual desire or thoughts? I suppose it might have been. We were basically just very good friends. But then again, thinking about it and looking at the logical side of it, that we were always together and that we hardly ever got into arguments, I reckon there was still something special in our relationship, and that we were doing fairly well.

Since I was experiencing these new and challenging psychological sides of epilepsy, the physical side did not change much. The frequency, type and intensity of my epileptic seizures pretty much remained as it was before the incident.

Chapter ten

I was getting in contact with quite a number of old acquaintances from my highschool days. It was also getting close to 20 years since I left South Africa, and therefore it was that long since I had finished school.

Then, one day, one of my Facebook friends sent me a link for an event that was due to take place in London. Somebody was organising a 20 year reunion for people from my final year at school - the 'matric year' as they call it in South Africa - for those who had moved to Europe. This sounded quite exciting. When I mentioned it to Bina, her first reaction was, "When are you leaving?", or in other words, "Oh wow! Of-course you're going."

We were in that position again, whereby I had the chance of going somewhere and would be away for a couple of days, apart from any close acquaintances. And the common thoughts, which always came to mind, "I hope I'll be OK" and "What if... ?".

I wasn't particularly over-excited at first. But as I started finding out which of my highschool friends had in fact moved to Europe, it changed everything. Most of them had moved to the UK. I was especially surprised to find out that three people from my 'matric' class had in fact moved to England.

Now I was really looking forward to this trip and I was making plans well in advance regarding where and when I would meet people. So, even though the main event, the reunion, was going to take place on the Friday evening, even before I left home I knew what I was going to be doing on some of the other days of the week.

The day of my trip to London had finally arrived. Even before I arrived at the hostel where I was going to spend the week, I had already been on the phone to one of my good best friends, Michael. He was one of my best friends from my highschool days and I couldn't believe that we would be meeting again. Before we got together I went out to see a bit of London. Everything was so different compared to Slovenia, the people, the atmosphere, everything. It was a place where I felt so much more comfortable.

I had decided to stay in a hostel as it was not only cheaper but I thought I would have a beter chance of meeting other people from all over the world. I actually met people from every continent of the world.

I met up with Michael and other school friends in the evenings, so I tended to spend the rest of the day out in London. Sometimes I even went around with other people from the hostel. In particular, there were two student pilots from Germany that I spent quite a lot of time with. We spoke a lot since I had also studied aeronautical engineering, so we had a lot to talk about. Then there was one other guy from South Africa I met, and a couple of other interesting people. I was being a lot more sociable than I had ever been in Slovenia. But one of the climaxes of my trip to London was the time I spent with Michael and some of his colleagues from work. I even surprised myself.

Then came the evening of the reunion. I can remember it so clearly, when I arrived at the restaurant where we planned to meet. I arrived a little early, and while waiting for the others to arrive I got a call from one of them saying they were not so sure if they'd be able to make it. While talking on the phone, one of the others arrived. It might have been 20 years, but the face in front of me was so familiar and I knew straight away who it was. We all had an amazing evening together.

In the last couple of days that I spent in London, I met a student from Spain. We spent some time, strolling through

London, chatting about all kinds of things. I shared quite a bit with her about my experiences from the last couple of years, and she also told me a lot about the experiences and challenges she had faced in recent years. We spoke about many different things, some even more emotional topics.

In conclusion, the time I spent in London was just amazing. There were experiences that entirely filled the week, and which also filled me with a great amount of positive energy. But it had obviously, and unfortunately, come to an end.

I was fortunate that I didn't have any problems at all at any time throughout the whole week. Not a single one, not even minor aura feelings. I just made sure that I took my medication and avoided those things that I knew could potentially cause problems, which was not at all difficult to do.

It was only after I returned home, back to the normal atmosphere, surroundings and tempo of life, that I started to notice differences and changes in my feelings. It was a great deal of those feelings that I so dearly missed and had been searching for so deeply in the last few years, and which were now, eventually, coming back to me. Including the feelings I had for Bina.

I simply couldn't understand why this was happening now. What was the reason that these feelings were only now coming back to me? Even though I had been trying so hard to find them and 'place them back', to get them back into my life, as with so many of the other feelings which did come back, Why?

It was more than four years since the incident by the school which had brought all this into my life. And only now was I managing to find some of those missing pieces, those missing feelings. Those vital and valuable parts of my psyche that were eventually returning back into my life. And only now, as everything was coming back, did I realise the full and complete extent of what was missing.

Since it was almost four-and-a-half years since the incident by the school, it wasn't as simple as just picking up the pieces and moving on. I would have very much liked it if it could have been as simple as that.

I had also noticed and felt strongly that for the whole four-and-a-half years Bina had practically been without a husband.

Whenever I tried to bring up the topic, Bina would always show some sort of dissatisfaction and wouldn't want to talk about it. This just showed me what she must have been feeling and experiencing the whole time, and what she must have gone through. But I still couldn’t understand. Why only now? After all this time and after all the effort I had put into it, why were these feelings coming back only now? I had so many unanswered questions.

I knew that because I had had such an excellent and social time in London, that it must have obviously had something to do with it.

Every bit of progress and change has its associated questions. Well, at least this time it did. I had so many unanswered questions. But I tried to take this step as I had with all of the rest - one step at a time. I would have to give it enough time and effort to pick up all the pieces.

One part of my psyche which had also been missing the whole time was physical, or rather sexual attraction, thoughts or feelings. Since the incident, and up until now, there had been absolutely none of these thoughts or feelings. Not in my thoughts, not anywhere. When I think about it, I noticed that when I was in London maybe those feelings of attraction had started coming back, but in such small amounts that I didn't really take much notice of them.

It was in those last couple of days that I was in London when I met the student from Spain. When I came home, I easily and freely told Bina about her. All I felt at that time was the possible development of a good friendship. These were the first signs that there was a part of my social psyche returning to my life. To me it was a good and welcome sign, s sign worth mentioning.

As so many of these pieces were now returning, I realised and started thinking more and more about how it must have been for Bina this whole time. As I started noticing these feelings and parts again, as they were slowly returning into my life, one after the other, I spent an increasing amount of time thinking about them.

I tried more and more often to talk to Bina about it, but she showed very little or no desire to talk about anything. I felt as if she clearly didn't want to reawaken those memories, or something. The memories of what had been going on in the last four years of our lives. So, I too eventually also stopped trying. This only showed me how much more difficult and unpleasant it really must have been for her.

What also returned was the natural sexual attraction, thoughts, or whatever you want to call it, I as a man sometimes had when I saw a woman. I felt a bit like a teenager again. But, to be honest with you, this was something I didn't particularly want back in my life, irrelevant of whatever some people may say; it's totally natural to have these thoughts. I preferred it when I had more pure, respectful feelings and thoughts about women, irrelevant of how they were dressed or how appealing they may have been. I felt as if I had this new feeling that was now contradicting those feelings of respect I had gained for women.

Another thought which kind of plagued my mind was what Bina must have thought when I had no sexual desire or temptation for her. I had thoughts like, "The only time a man would ever be like this to his wife would be if he had a lover i.e. if he was cheating on her".

I would have so much liked to just pick up the pieces and carry on from this point. But it wasn't that simple. This was an area where both of our feelings were involved, not only mine. Not only my 'lost' feelings and lost psyche, but also Bina's damaged feelings. I was totally aware that was something which had been going on for quite a number of years.

Even though there were so many parts of my psyche returning to my life, I still didn't feel like the same person I was before the incident. Even though I had made so much progress in so many areas of my psyche, I still felt different and incomplete.

The desire to socialise was still minimal, if at all. I was just lucky that I had so many other things to do, which kept me and my mind busy, so that I wouldn't think too much about what was still missing and incomplete.

One new addition was that I started spending an increasing amount of time pursuing my interest in epilepsy. Now, as I felt I was making more and more progress myself, I spent more time reading about epilepsy. Sometimes, when I had a check-up, I also shared and discussed some of those findings, which pertained closely to my condition, with my neurologist. I found quite a few interesting articles and papers about various studies that had been done on patients with epilepsy.

One of those articles was a very interesting and extensive article about the effects of Coca-Cola on the body, and the reaction it has with the main contents of the medication I was taking, 'tegretol', or ’carbamazepine’ as it is known in the medical world. I didn't really take that much notice of it and didn’t want to really believe it at first, because of all the other negative rumours and side effects one would so often hear about Coca-Cola.

But then one day Timmy and I were in a large shopping centre in the city. We were alone when those aura feelings came along. They became quite strong and unpleasant, which made me really worried. It was at such an inappropriate moment, when I was alone with Timmy. At the same time Timmy asked if we could get something to drink so I decided, "OK!, I'll have a Coke to see if it really helps". As soon as I took a gulp or two of Coke, the feelings disappeared almost instantly and I felt perfectly alright after that. It was so rare that I felt so good after feeling such aura effects, like the ones I experienced that day in the shopping centre. This was a clear indication to me that there absolutely must be some truth in the article that I had read.

After the experience in the shopping centre, I did more research on the effects of Coca-Cola. When I found out who actually invented Coca-Cola - a pharmacist who was better known as a doctor, and his main initial intention of the drink - it was then a lot easier to believe the contents of the article I had found.

If you do a bit of research on what the native Americans used the original ingredients of Coca-Cola for, you will soon believe me! How the contents of the cola nut, when chewed, strengthen and heal the digestive system, and the cola leaves when chewed, heal and strengthen muscle problems. Adding the other ingredients found in Coca-Cola, it became the first energy drink and was used for many ailments.

I shared this information with my neurologist and after a short review on his computer, he too confirmed what I said about the article; about the combination between the main contents of my medication, carbamazepine, and the characteristics and effects of Coca-Cola.

Coca-Cola is used by professional cyclists during long cycling stages as an energy enhancer. It enhances energy levels and the caffeine keeps them stable for a lengthened time. Finding this out only made it even more interesting to read about. It's these unusual characteristics of Coca-Cola, exploited by cyclists, which also makes it beneficial for people suffering from epilepsy. It's the caffeine, which is so often condemned that is actually beneficial for the body.

Later I noticed something which additionally supported and practically confirmed that Coca-Cola could in fact be beneficial for people suffering from epilepsy. If we look at the effects of Coca-Cola on the body, it can be seen how it enhances and stabilises energy levels in the body. This is almost the opposite of how the body reacts to carbohydrates. Here we are practically covering the main attributes of diets used to combat epilepsy in youth.

This experience only showed me the value of information one can find. Information which is out there just waiting to be found, used, and manipulated by anybody willing to search for it.

Well there you go. I actually 'tasted' for myself the value and benefits of the time spent on the internet. Reading all kinds of stuff about all these different topics associated with epilepsy. For once I noticed the time I spent on the internet reading about epilepsy definitely hadn't gone to waste. It actually contributed to more than just enriching my knowledge, for once it also had practical benefits.

Chapter eleven

I started reading quite a lot. Feeding my interest and curiosity about various topics and areas associated with epilepsy. I realised that there is actually quite a lot one can find on the internet about epilepsy. You just need to have a bit of an idea what to look for.

Since I was now also interested in the psychological aspects of epilepsy, such as the 'psychosocial disorder', I had so much more to search for and to read about. I was well aware of what had happened to me and of what was going on with me the whole time.

All this curiosity and interest obviously also helped me understand and cope a lot more easily with what I was facing and going through. I started learning a lot, especially about myself and from my personal experiences.

I was also honoured and privileged to eventually meet two people who were in the rescue team that had rescued me off the mountain that day. But how we came in touch with each other was entirely coincidental. Interestingly it was through my children, Sarah and Timmy, that I came in touch with them. It was through general conversation and chatting. The conversation apparently went in such a direction that my accident was mentioned and enough was said for them to realise, "Hey, I remember that, I was there!"

Firstly, I was amazed that Sarah's grade two teacher was among the group. It was actually quite special when I found this out, because about the only thing I remembered about being in the helicopter was a woman's voice keeping me calm.

The second rescuer we met was through the climbing club that Timmy attended. Timmy even had the chance to go climbing in the Slovenian Alps with this individual, so they were in quite regular contact with each other. He was quite active in the climbing community in general and was also a mountain rescuer.

I was incredibly curious about how he still remembered me and my accident after such a long time, after twenty years. Even though the mountain rescue team deals with quite a number of rescues each year, he still remembered my incident. When I spoke to him I asked him how, or why, he remember me, to which he replied, “You always remember the incidents with more serious injuries”. He described one other similar incident that he was involved in. An incident where the person had obtained more serious injuries than I had. He concluded that it’s always nice to know that the person survived and has recovered from his/her injuries.

It was nice to meet and to get to know both of them, and to hear their opinions and comments as members of the mountain rescue team.

I started taking more notice of other people, their feelings and what may be going on in their minds. Some of the images and quotes people were placing and sharing in the media, is one place where this was most noticeable. Sometimes they would really grab my attention and also get me pondering over the full and deeper meaning of the quotes or texts. I sometimes even wondered why this particular friend was placing such expressions and the message behind what they were sharing.

Then it happened. I noticed a post, a message, which one of my friends put on Facebook. It was unusual that she started placing such messages; I clearly saw and felt that something must be wrong. The messages her posts were conveying were clearly saying something to me. I don't remember what it was in particular, but I reached out and sent her a message.

We started communicating and exchanging messages more regularly. After a couple of messages, she felt comfortable enough to open up to me more and explain what she was going through. She was having quite a few personal issues that were causing her a lot of emotional pain.

I suppose it was from my personal experience and from all the reading I was doing about the 'psychosocial disorder' and similar issues, that I noticed something was wrong in the way she was expressing herself on Facebook. I also got that feeling that she might be alone in these challenges.

When this friend felt that she could explain what it was, what she was going through, it touched me even more. It was in those areas of my feelings, emotions and mentality where I had gained so much respect for women. Or in other words, the respect I had gained for the mothers of all children. It was in this part of life where this friend was suffering the most.

After we had been in touch for some time, and after sharing a lot of my opinions and experiences with her, she said to me that I should definitely go out and share my way of thinking and my mentality with people, because "there are many people out there who need to hear what you have to say", she added. She obviously noticed and liked my way of thinking and how I expressed myself.

This friend concluded that I had made a really big difference to the way she faced her challenges and how she was thinking and facing all that was going on in her life at that moment. "It would be wrong to keep this to yourself", she concluded. Her reaction touched me so much and made me realise the value of the positive way of thinking that I strived to follow. I helped her see a light at the end of a very dark tunnel, which obviously made me feel pretty good too.

I was really glad that I was able to comfort somebody who simply needed someone to listen and understand what she was experiencing. This really meant a lot to me because I was able to make a difference in an area of life and emotion where I myself was suffering.

As I was pondering over the challenges other people were facing, it helped put my challenges in a different perspective. It was obvious that my condition and my challenges had changed me as a person. It never occurred to me that my way of thinking and the way I had chosen to face my challenges would ever be of interest to others.

In early 2014 I was scheduled to spend a week in hospital. They wanted to do a week-long brain scan, or EEG (electroencephalography), as it is otherwise called. All I really had to do was to just be there connected to the apparatus.

The goal in doing a week-long scan was to get as much information as possible, while awake, while sleeping and at various stages throughout the day. A great amount of information can be obtained if a person has a seizure while being scanned. For this reason, I was taken off medication, yet still I didn’t have any seizures.

There wasn’t much for me to do at the hospital, since Bina and the kids could come only for about an hour or so per day. And considering that I am not much of a ‘book worm’, it meant that keeping myself busy in that way also wasn't much of an option. Thus, it didn't take long before I started getting into conversations with other patients and with various personnel at the clinic, those who specialise in various fields of neurology, not only in epilepsy. There were also medical students doing various tasks in the clinic. Talking with all these people brought up some interesting conversations.

Towards the end of the week spent in the clinic, I met a neurologist with whom I had some interesting and quite extensive conversations. At one stage his reaction to one of my comments made quite an impression. A reaction I will never forget. We spoke about topics that I had been giving quite some thought to while in the clinic. While chatting to other patients in the clinic, I started wondering whether perhaps epileptic seizures don't always originate in the brain.

I was also giving much thought to the EEG scan. When I explained my various opinions to the neurologist, he replied to one of my thoughts "Well, that's quite interesting, I have never really given much thought to that", or something like that. For me to get such a reply from a neurologist, or in other words from someone specialising in this field, really made a big impression.

Because of the reaction and comments I received from the specialist in the clinic, I took some time and combined some of my opinions and information I found on the internet about the topic, and united them in a short paper. After about a week I had to return to the clinic, so I decided to take the 'paper' with me to give to my specialist, so he could read it - if he was able to find the time. My specialist is a very social doctor, always prepared to listen and chat about what I, the patient, had to say, or to ask.

About a week or two after I was in the clinic, I had another check-up with my neurologists. It was almost like a summary of the results of the scan and the reports written by the doctors while I was in the clinic. Since I hadn't had any epileptic seizures while being scanned, the results of the scan didn't give as much information as they would have, if I had a seizure during the process. My neurologist recommended that it could be wise to repeat the week-long scan in the hope of getting better results.

Towards the end of the check-up we spoke a little about the paper which I had put together and had given him to read. He was quite impressed and even asked me for permission to use the contents of the paper.

My neurologist's comments made quite a big impression on me. We then spoke about getting involved. He gave me information about a local organisation, the LIGA against epilepsy Slovenia, which is involved in the epilepsy community. Not only did this make a big impression, but it obviously also greatly affected my self-esteem and self-worth, which was also suffering greatly.

I got in contact with the organisation, the LIGA, and they invited me to come to the next event which they were planning to hold in a neighbouring city. I warmly accepted the invitation. I even had the idea and took on the challenge of going to this event by bike. It was in a city about 65km from my home. It was a bit of a challenge cycling there, but I enjoyed the trip. I obviously made quite an impression on a number of people, particularly by coming so far by bike. Even on the leadership of the organisation. They even let me introduce myself, since it was the first time I had ever been to such an event held by this organisation. I remained in contact with the LIGA, got to know them a little better, and they got to know me too.

It was turning out to be quite an active year for me. Firstly, the incident with my friend on Facebook, then the conversations I had with various personnel and with my specialist at the clinic and then finally, getting in contact with the LIGA. This made me feel good about myself, getting out and being a bit more social. Up till now I had been leading quite a narrow-minded kind of life, not getting 'out and around' or socialising much at all.

I don't know how much all this change and activity, physical and social, was affecting the seizures I was having. But I noticed and had a feeling that the 'shape' or kind of seizures I was having were changing.

Firstly, there was the one experience when I had a seizure outside while cycling. This was unusual, since I had never, or very rarely, had seizures outside, and secondly I had never had them when I was being physically active, such as cycling. This was really unusual. What I did notice though, was that by the time the paramedics arrived, I had more or less come back to my senses. It was unusual for me to be 'up and running' so soon after having a seizure.

Later I found the possible reason why the seizure could have happened, and why outside. That day I was taking it slowly and was pretty much lazing around. I still remember so clearly how I had been lazing on the couch when I decided to go cycling. I believe that because I put my body through too much of a physical change in such a short time, that must surely have had something to do with it. I once again went onto the internet and found articles and various texts which supported the idea that too much change in too short a space of time is not good.

Then there were a couple of other seizures that followed. They were all similar to that first one when I felt that I came back to my senses quite quickly and I didn't have all those problems, headaches etc. that I normally had after having a seizure. This led to the question; "Are my seizures changing to lighter ones"?

Then there was a second seizure that again occurred outside while I was on my bike, i.e. while being physically active. Only this time it happened in the morning while going to work.

This was most unusual, because I had never had seizures in the mornings. And again, a seizure outside.

Then, once again, I began searching for the reason for that seizure. When I look back, I noticed I had made two mistakes that day. I woke, got ready and headed off on my way to work as usual. However, the first mistake was that I normally took a snack with me so I could eat it at work. The second, as had been the case with the previous seizure, was that I had done everything too quickly. I woke up, got washed and dressed, grabbed my backpack and headed off. All in a matter of 15 minutes or so.

To prevent this from happening again, all I did was to add breakfast to my morning schedule. It was also very interesting that when I went back to the lady who noticed me and who then called the ambulance, she said that I was just standing there in her driveway, looking lost. She knew that something was not right, so she called for an ambulance. What was unusual is that the lady found me just standing there, and secondly I didn't have any bumps or bruises as a result of the events of that day. Was this all pointing to the fact and the possibility that I hadn't fallen down?

It was also these few incidents, in a reasonably short time, which made a real impression on my interest in epilepsy, and also, if not more so, on the way I chose to face the challenges of having the condition. This gave me the inspiration to continue widening my interest in epilepsy. I realised that I could maybe take all this desire and interest and put it to some good, positive use. Who knows, maybe I could even help other people in similar situations to mine.

Additionally, I also came to realise that I can almost always find the reason why the seizure happened.

I always had that thought, "Well, I am an engineer, specialised in a field far from health and neurology, so what could I do or say that would be of interest to anybody else." Well, I was now finding out and realised that maybe I was wrong.

But one of the greater attributes or characteristics of epilepsy is that there is so much an individual can themselves implement into their lifestyles to make their own lives better. Changes that each individual can easily and freely introduce by themselves to help cope more easily with the challenges of having and living with the condition.

It was this characteristic of epilepsy that drew my attention and interest. In time, it was this that formed the backbone of the person I became, that my health and wellbeing is also dependent on what I put into it. I was surprised by how much each individual can themselves do to help cope a little more easily with the condition. Even though it is such a dynamic and sensitive condition.

While studying and reading about all the different sides and topics of epilepsy that I had become interested in, I came across a whole amount of other documents and papers about various other sides of it.

What interests me most are papers that cover observations and tests made by specialists. What is most interesting are the statistical results, explanations for those results, and the possible reasons for any fluctuations. A great deal of what I read and found, also became the foundations of a number of the changes I implemented into my own lifestyle.

One other value of all this reading and statistical information I had found was that I was noticing how and what other people with epilepsy were dealing with their condition and how it influenced their own lives. Or rather, from a more psychological point of view, what people weren't doing! And how people were being psychologically affected by the condition by not doing certain things. For instance, how people were simply allowing the condition to take them over and take away their freedom. There are so many examples of how people practically shut themselves off from the outside world. This was the common factor that I had not only read about, but had also felt and experienced in my own life. So I said to myself, "This is definitely not the way I want to go!".

With all the reading and studying I was doing, I started to notice the many different faces of epilepsy. But, on the other hand, being so different and individual, epilepsy also has common characteristics. Characteristics that were being affected by some of the various implementations I was introducing into my own lifestyle.

This made me slowly realise the value of all the reading and studying I was doing. The value of the information I was obtaining. In the end, I realised that even though I am an engineer by profession, far from any medical calling, I was still noticing and finding a great deal of information that I felt that people needed to know, but are not getting.

What made me even more surprised was that I was finding all this interesting and valuable information about how I can make my life better and even combat epilepsy, but I had never noticed any information or anything relating to this in any clinics or hospitals. I only found all this information because I had such a strong desire and interest to search for it. This also gave me more strength and desire to talk about it.

I was still living quite a narrow-minded lifestyle. Not socialising much at all. Well, a lot less than practically everybody else around me. What was interesting, though, was that I preferred being in the presence of strangers or with people I barely knew, rather than being with people I knew well.

Even while cycling I had quite a number of interesting experiences. Cycling is actually quite a social sport. Cyclists often greet each other when they cross paths and it is quite common to get into conversations with other cyclists when you stop at a common resting place.

I often pondered over the reason for this. For not feeling too comfortable being with common acquaintances, and even relatives. What I knew for certain was that I definitely didn't like how so many people were always so clever and always thought they knew what was best for me, especially when it came to comments and suggestions about my health and my condition. If they knew somebody, or had somebody close to them, who also suffered from epilepsy, then OK! Maybe then they may have something beneficial or wise to say, but otherwise?

What I found interesting were the statistics about how people with epilepsy were doing exactly the opposite. How they rather avoided contact with the general public. Maybe it was because I was acquainted with this fact, that, in my sub-conscious, I was putting effort into being different and trying to be more sociable.

One day all of these features of being more communicative, easily conversing with strangers, and meeting foreigners, all came together. Well, actually, this kind of thing happened quite a number of times, but this time it was going to turn out to be quite unique.

I was in the nearby grocery store when I noticed two foreigners at the bread counter. I assumed they needed a little help communicating with the baker behind the counter, so I gladly stepped in and offered my assistance.

They actually didn't need help. They were at the shop together with their son, who lives in Kamnik and is familiar with the language. It was great as it meant that at least I had found another foreigner living here. This was really nice, since I so much enjoyed meeting foreigners, and now there was one living nearby.

We met a couple of times. Took slow strolls through town, chatting. It didn't take long for me to get on to the topic of my condition. We spoke a bit about the epilepsy I have, how it came to be that I have it, and so on. I got so far and explained how I have accepted living with the condition and the challenges of living with epilepsy. I explained that I am comfortable with it and can easily talk about the condition and how it affects my life.

It is more common that people with epilepsy hardly ever want to talk about their condition. Not me, or at least, not anymore. I am pretty comfortable about it and not at all embarrassed that I have it. I also mentioned that I was looking into the idea of getting involved in the epilepsy community.

That was when this new friend mentioned how he was in contact with a neurologist who is writing a book about epilepsy and wanted to publish it in English too. It didn't take long for me to meet the neurologist. He actually recognised me from the event that had taken place some weeks before that I had decided to cycle to. We met a number of times after that and had some interesting discussions. It turned out that he also works in conjunction with the LIGA against epilepsy I had met.

This was just one of those unique incidents, which came as a result of me not being embarrassed about my condition.

Then, on another occasion I was chatting to a friend I had met through the sports community. We didn't really know each other that well, so he was quite surprised when I mentioned that I suffer from epilepsy. We spoke a little about it and I explained what it is like, how it influences life and how it feels living with the condition. That was when he mentioned some concerns they were having about their daughter.

He explained how his daughter had these moments of being unresponsive and seems as if she was daydreaming or something. At first I was unsure, but it sounded a little like it could be a light form of epilepsy, commonly known as absence, if anything at all. But obviously, I'm no specialist so I am always cautious before jumping to any conclusions. My friend said that they had mentioned this to their daughter's doctor, but she said there's most probably nothing wrong and they need not worry.

Then, a couple of days later, we ran into each other again. He now had a recording of his daughter while having one of these spells. It was while she was playing and being active. After watching the video recording and seeing her having one of these spells, I strongly recommended they see a doctor and get a referral to see a specialist about it, which they also did. They got a referral to see a neurologist.

This friend contacted me after they had had the check-up, with very good and surprising news. Firstly, when he mentioned me to the neurologist and said that I had recommended they see a specialist, the neurologist replied that he had actually heard of me, WOW! And secondly, it was a good idea that they had been for the check-up and scan, because they indeed did notice some interference in her brain function. They were very lucky to have found this now because it meant it was much easier and better to treat the condition while she was still so young before it developed into a more difficult to treat condition.

In just a few years, my life had taken a number of complete turnarounds. And, more than once, they were like complete head-over-heels flips. But what I was about to realise is that I had landed on much more solid and more sturdy ground. Where was this leading? From all that I had lost and after all that had happened to me. Where was this going? How far was this going to go?

Chapter twelve

It was those few specific and unique incidents that gave me the desire and that extra self-confidence and self-esteem to get up and act. But, most of all, these incidents showed me that I could actually do something, and not only for myself. It was true that I was in contact with the LIGA organisation already, but now I felt that I could really get actively involved and actually make a difference for other people too.

What was also great was that I was at least getting in contact with more and more people and I was being more social. Additionally, I was now meeting many other people who were facing the same challenges of living with epilepsy as I was, which I hadn't ever done before. My life was going through another one of those changes, another one of those 'steps of progress'. Well, that was how I felt about myself.

Not only was I getting to know the LIGA organisation and the people better, but they were getting to know me too. I went there reasonably regularly and it didn't take long for me to realise that there was no active support group in the area, so I put forward a suggestion to create one.

I was definitely 'getting out and around' more and more. I was now facing head on the one challenge that I had been having such great difficulty with - being sociable and fitting in. This one issue had always caused so much emotional pain because it was something I really wanted and needed, but simply couldn’t get.

It was good that I was getting out more, as it meant that I spent less time thinking about myself and my condition. Even though I was still thinking about epilepsy, I wasn’t getting stressed and over-exaggerating about my condition, as so many people with epilepsy do. I’m sure the atmosphere and direction of my thoughts also had a positive influence. Even though I was thinking so much more about epilepsy, my thoughts were about cures and solutions for the condition.

Since I was now coming in contact with other people, who, like me, were facing the same challenges of suffering with epilepsy, I became even more comfortable with it.

I will never forget the initial comment of one of the doctors, who, right at the beginning when I had barely got to know the LIGA, said that it would be a good idea for me to get more involved in sports and recreation for people suffering from epilepsy. He noticed how physically active I was. So, I put an idea forward to hold a recreational day in Kamnik, the town where I lived. Since Kamnik is always so active and alive with regular activities and events, I thought it would be an ideal location for such an event. They warmly welcomed the suggestion.

Now I was really getting involved. First with the support group, and now with this recreational event. This only increased the desire and the passion to study epilepsy even more. I even went as far as purchasing books. Because I felt and found out the value and importance of nutrition on general wellbeing, especially for those suffering from epilepsy, the books were based on the effects of nutrition on the brain.

Since I was quite comfortable talking with strangers, meeting new people and other patients through the LIGA organisation, it was easy and I became even more comfortable talking about it and with the fact that I myself suffer from it. It was also a lot easier to talk to strangers who were suffering the same challenges as I was, than it was to talk with closer friends or relatives. Simply because other people who don't know anything about epilepsy, didn't really understand how I was feeling. Talking to other people about epilepsy also made it a lot easier for me to face the condition.

I had some really unique experiences with some of the people I met. One experience in particular, which made a big impression, was a lady who came to the LIGA organisation. Her seizures had become so regular that it was greatly influencing her life. What she missed most was the ability to be able to freely spend quality time with her children. It was fortunate that she came that day, because she and her husband were the only ones who turned up that day, so we were alone. While talking with her and while sharing experiences with each other, I noticed a couple of things in her general way of life, things which I had changed in mine. One was the importance and effects nutrition has on general wellbeing. So, I recommended that she try to make some changes to her diet.

After getting in touch with her a short while after we met and spoke for the first time, she said that she had felt such a dramatic improvement in her wellbeing. And then, a couple of months later, we were in touch with each other again. I found out that the frequency of her seizures had in fact dropped by an amazing 97%. From about three to four seizures per week, to about one seizure every two months. It was more than just a change in the amount of seizures she was having. She felt as if she had got her life back. These kinds of experiences make all that time, effort and study of epilepsy so worthwhile, lift me up and really 'makes my day'.

But, as I was eventually getting 'out and about' more, I was going through some more changes. Changes which greatly influenced me on the 'inside'. Those parts of my 'insides', of my feelings and emotions, which were all so influenced, damaged and practically ripped away from me. I was developing and rebuilding up my self-worth and self-esteem.

I don't know how this, if at all, was influencing my seizures. But I also experienced a change there too. I experienced a period when I barely had any aura's, not even light ones. And furthermore, I even went through a period where I had six months between seizures. There was only once when I had such a long time between them. It was when I introduced omega-3 oil into my diet.

Then there were those periods when I would have seizures barely a few months apart. These kinds of experiences only upset me, just when I was thinking that there might eventually be some more progress, or some change. This was a warning, "Not so quick!".

Since coming in contact with the organisation, LIGA against epilepsy - meeting doctors, psychiatrists and other people who specialised in various fields in the medical world - and additionally meeting with all these other people, who were also suffering from epilepsy, it became something quite unique and special. It opened so many new doors into my life.

With all these changes and bits of progress I was making, I felt it in my psyche, and in my confidence and self-worth. I took it one step further and took on one big new challenge.

I might have been getting involved and getting to know people better, and spending a lot more time on other people. But all this effort, all this work and involvement, was really about me. I was opening all these new 'doors'. Doors to my insides, doors to my psyche, doors to my heart. These were some of those many doors, which were practically slammed in my face as a result of the incident in 2008 and what followed in the few years after that. Or were these doors that I was now opening for the first time, I don't know?

The incident of December 2008 was now quite far behind me. The psychological recovery was a long one and a constant never-ending challenge and never-ending journey. Or would it be better to say, a "never-ending story", since it wasn't simply a journey to find myself again, but you might rather say, an interesting exploration. It was a great deal more than that; it was more like a never-ending adventure, to find myself again.

Whenever I reached such stages where I was making new and major progress, I often asked myself, "Is this it, is this the person I have become?". I knew and was well aware what was missing in my life. I put a great deal of effort into recovering from all that I had lost: physically, psychologically, everything. But mostly psychologically.

As time went on, and as more and more of these steps of recovery and progress were now behind me, I became aware that I had come a long way and that I had pretty much recovered from my whole ordeal. But this only made me think even further. I was well aware of the many things I had lost and what was still possibly missing in my life. I knew I still had issues I needed to work on and I constantly did so, to become even better and stronger. Since I had come so far, I started raising new questions.

I always knew and felt what was missing in life. I knew what challenges I had, and worked to overcome them. That was how I had come so far and defeated many of those challenges that I had had up until now. In many aspects, I was pretty content and satisfied with the person I was becoming. It was important to me to become the best person I possibly could.

But one big question still remained! Were there maybe issues that I perhaps didn't realise or take notice of? Issues that were no longer in my mind or psyche. Issues that maybe people around me, the people closest to me, were noticing and were still missing, but not mentioning?

Chapter thirteen

Life is filled with all kinds of issues: adventures, challenges, unique experiences, ... It's a clear sign that life is actually going somewhere, that it's moving forward. It means a lot to me to have that feeling, that confirmation of progress, that life actually is going somewhere. And that is also how I generally felt, that life is indeed moving forward.

It all relates back to that day, back in 2011, when I decided, "NO, I'm not going to allow this to take over my life and bring me down" and, "this is not the way I want to go on anymore".

I was extremely proud and happy that I had created a foundation and that I had stuck to it. A foundation on to which I was able to build the greater part of the person I had become. I strongly believe that this had a great influence on some of those unique experiences I had, and also on the decisions I was making. Like the one to start working with the organisation, 'LIGA against epilepsy'. It had become a foundation I could strongly lean on.

It was a foundation that guided and directed me to reach heights I previously could not and did not reach. Heights I never knew I could reach. Higher than I had ever before, higher than I could have imagined.

Even though I was still facing some serious and difficult challenges on the way, such as my marriage, I had this foundation which slowly but surely started supporting me and the challenges I was facing. I was also noticing how I was changing because of it, the way I started to look at and face challenges and life in general. This only showed me how strong this foundation was actually becoming.

I was rebuilding my life, trying to place as much as I could on this foundation. It wasn't always easy and I knew it wouldn't be, to build myself back up. Logically, it often became more challenging. Even though I was becoming stronger and even though I had become more aware of feelings: my feelings and those of others. I was now putting more emphasis on those feelings; I could place them all on this foundation. But this foundation supported more than just feelings. A lot more!

One such place where I felt my strength come out was in my cycling. Cycling was something I started at an early age, and it's something I have stuck with. But now I felt that I was actually stepping it up, higher and much more than ever before. Even though my prime years as a sportsman were now well behind me and I was facing this condition straight in the face, I was still reaching heights and capabilities with my cycling, which surprised me. Cycling influenced me everywhere: my physical wellbeing of course, but also areas not associated so much with riding my bike, such as my sensitivity and my emotions.

Since I had become more social with other cyclists, I had got to know quite a number of them who lived in the same town as I did. I quite often crossed paths with them while in town and I would often get into interesting conversations about cycling.

Then there were those people who were active in the organisation committee for the local triathlon team in which I was also actively involved.

It was nice being with these people, who all emit such positive, encouraging and enthusiastic energy. It was no wonder that some of them were so active and successful in their individual sports categories. This also started to rub off on me. It was closely related to that optimism I had put so much emphasis on and it certainly also helped it grow like it did.

This optimism definitely played a part in me being able to slowly and comfortably go beyond anything I had ever been capable of doing before. Not that I previously wasn't able to, but I had no such desire or inspiration to go so far. Not that I had that desire or a set goal to go so far now, but I simply went as far as I comfortably wanted to and felt I could. The height, the level that I was now able to reach was so much higher than it had ever been before. Was this partially as a result of the way I had decided to aim my life? I most certainly think it had a significant part to play. It was a clear indication that I could actually see and feel.

It didn't take long before people started encouraging me and asking why I don't take part in any of the local cycling events and competitions.

I had never really ever thought of the idea of taking part in any competitive cycling events. I'm not a competitive type of cyclist, more a recreational one. What was also holding me back was that I was aware of how taking part in competitive sports could actually induce epileptic seizures. But as I was becoming more tempted and encouraged to take part, I did more research on the subject. What I found out didn't really deter me. I also fortunate that to live in a period where physical activity and taking part in sports is actually being more encouraged for many health conditions in general. So, finding information was not at all difficult. There is an abundance of inspirational information, and one can easily find concrete information and results of studies done by specialists on the subject. In the past, people suffering from almost any health condition were more than discouraged from taking part in almost any physical activity or sport.

The date of a popular annual cycling marathon, which started and ended in my home town, was getting closer. So, there was obviously a lot of talk about it going on, and some of the people I knew were encouraging me to join them. So, I did exactly that and decided, “Heck, let’s go for it!”.

It was a really brave and somewhat scary decision to make, because I was about to sign up for the most challenging marathon of the cycling season in Slovenia. It is a little over 130km and over 2000m of climbing hills over the Alps, into Austria and back into Slovenia.

At first, as the marathon was getting closer, I had feelings such as, “What am I getting myself into?” But as time went on and as the marathon got closer and closer, I became more and more enthusiastic and was looking forward to it.

When the day finally arrived, the preparations were all complete and as cyclists started assembling in the town centre, the magnitude of the event became evident. I had watched the marathon in previous years, but always from the sidelines. Now I was actually in it. I decided I would rather start towards the back, rather than being in the main pack. The feeling and elation was really something. As I was well into the marathon and we were heading into the Alps, I noticed that I was going much faster and better than I normally ever could on my own. I believe it was the excitement, adrenaline and atmosphere of taking part that was pushing me to go so much faster. Was this that same effect that pushes many to go too far and to exceed their own physical capabilities? The effect that can be the cause of those ‘exercise induced seizures’ we hear so much about, for many suffering from epilepsy who have tried taking part in sports but experienced seizures whilst doing so. I was well aware of this and put a lot of emphasis into ensuring that I wouldn’t do the same.

I completed the marathon. I finished towards the back, where I had started. But I finished it! I felt like a winner.

But my cycling wasn't only about taking part and being active. There were some aspects of cycling that were greatly influencing me as a person. It was kind of like a two-way relationship. What you put in is what you get out, and more. A lot more!

I started to face my challenges differently and with more confidence. I started paying more attention to the destination, rather than to the journey. For instance, when I was cycling up a hilly section, I began paying more attention to the top of the hill, to the sunshine breaking through over the top of the hill, rather than on the road, to make it to the top. It made it easier to get to the top, well at least for me it did. I found that I started to use this method or tactic in more than just my cycling.

Cycling really showed me how I could go further; how to face challenges, how to take that step further, and how I could safely go further than I had ever intended or imagined I could. It showed me that I had more in myself than I had in my self-esteem.

If it wasn't for these positive sides of life, like these unique experiences and feelings of progress, getting through those moments of depression, downfalls and other more challenging parts of life would obviously have been so much more difficult, if not impossible.

It was and is this model that I had imagined and which I also share with many people. I imagine every situation in life as a handful full of pebbles. Nice and smooth ones, and rough, colourless ones. It's our personal decision which of these we are going to choose and take notice of: is it the rough negative ones, or the lovely smooth positive ones? It's all in front of us.

It was always nice to have, to be able to notice, and to be able to concentrate on these positive and optimistically encouraging factors, but it was obviously still often difficult due to the ever-present uninspiring and pessimistically orientated thoughts and challenges.

It was these experiences - both the difficult and the inspiring - that shaped me into the person I have become, which brought out my sensitivity, my vulnerability and especially, the level of respect I have for people.

One day all of these things that I had gained, a greater part of the person I had become, came together in one incident. I was on my way home on my bike, when I came upon a car accident that had just happened. There was little time to think, so I reacted and helped a lady who was injured in one of the cars. I will never forget the compliment the paramedics gave me when they arrived and took over.

But what was even more unbelievable was when I was helping out at a triathlon event almost a year later. A woman came up to me and asked if I was the one who helped out in an accident that happened almost a year ago. It's true that it was quite an incident to remember, especially for those involved, but I was still amazed that someone remembered me and what I did, and for so long. I didn't see my actions as anything 'special'. It was a clear sign of the person I was becoming, possibly someone worth remembering.

This was the person I had become and my life was constantly finding direction. But it was no longer just in some random direction as it might have been in the past. But it was a direction I was content with and wanted to continue in. I knew that the life in front of me would have its challenges, but then whose life doesn't? Challenges are all part of the progress and part of the growth. It just depends what we chose to do with them?

Chapter fourteen

Even though I was making some decent progress in one part of my life, I was still quite an unsociable and fairly introvert person. This was the side of me where I felt that I was becoming especially stronger, where I had felt exceptional growth and progress. I had become more expressionistic, I was more aware and took more notice of expressions and feelings. It was a unique part of the sensitive and emotional person I had become.

Those challenges and the so hard to find pieces of my feelings and emotions that were so altered, had become so sensitive and vulnerable. This only resulted in me having greater respect for those feelings and giving them deeper meaning. Not only for my own feelings, but also, if not more, respect for the feelings of others.

It is not only the visual expressions one gives out and sees, but more the message behind every expression and every image. It wasn't so much the expressions that I was giving out, but more the mood, the expressions and the messages that others were giving out, which I was starting to take more notice of. The story and message behind every image and every expression.

One place I really noticed this was in some of the images and quotes that people were placing and sharing on the web. They would sometimes really grab my attention and also get me thinking.

It's these values that have been with me since the early stages of my recovery. For instance, that 'message', that troubling atmosphere I noticed and felt in the posts my friend was placing on Facebook, which resulted in me reaching out and offering a word of support. That single event, which I believe played a big part in me becoming that much more sensitive, passionate and caring person that I have become.

And it was these values, these attributes, which were once again going to come out on top, above all others. It was another one of those posts in the media. A post placed by a friend on Facebook, like so many others. But this one post made such an exceptional impression on me. It was an expression which was quite relevant to me, my life and certain interests at that moment of time. It was a photo of a cyclist with a long straight road behind them. Along with the photo there was an expression, "I haven't come so far to only come so far!" I could so easily picture myself there, on that bike, on that long straight road. Saying exactly that! Even though I had come quite far and achieved so much in the last number of years, I felt that I still had a long way to go and that I had to keep going.

One issue which still so greatly suffered as a result of all the challenges and changes I had faced was my marriage. And since my marriage was so important and valuable to me, and also involved so much, these missing pieces were felt, missed and noticed so much more than so many others, which also made a great impression in life. Since my marriage and relationship with my wife involved so much - physically, psychologically, emotionally and more - it obviously suffered that much more. And since I felt that I was making progress, advances and change in general in life, here I had this one issue that was going almost nowhere. You can only imagine how that made me feel.

What I could never understand and what made me so much more upset, was how my feelings for my children did come back and had progressed so much, into something so special and so strong into something it had never been before and in a reasonably short time. But my marriage and my feelings for

Bina, what had happened to them, and why? Why was it so different and so much harder? WHY?

My marriage didn't have that long a road behind it like so many other issues did, because it simply didn't progress and recover as much as all those other parts of life had. And even after 2013, after I started taking more notice of emotions and feelings, and putting that much more efort into those sensitive issues, like my relationship with Bina, it still never really got back on track and never really recovered.

I know and understand that it must certainly have been difficult for Bina too, to have me the way I was. Especially in the period shortly after the incident, from 2009 all the way through 2013. But I also know and was well aware of the effort I was putting into our relationship. But still, it made such little progress. Why?

I found that my mind and my mood often lingered and I was edging away from the foundation I had created. Especially when I was thinking about my feelings and the challenges I was facing. There were times when the optimism I was putting so much effort and emphasis into, would linger and fall.

Obviously, it's normal that a person has their good and bad days. But whenever I thought more about myself and especially about my marriage and my relationship with Bina, then it often became a really sensitive moment for me. What made it worse was that I simply allowed it to continue affecting me so much. I didn't know otherwise. I was lost.

I often had that feeling that to Bina I was just a patient. She often showed concern over whether I was taking my medication and would often call me when I was running a bit late. Whether while I was out cycling or whatever, it didn't really matter? All she was interested was if I was OK. But she showed little or no interest in other relevant issues, such as my sensitive feelings or my emotions. Neither was there any interest in our relationship. That is the general impression and feeling I got from her of how it stood.

I knew that it was quite common with those suffering from epilepsy for their spouse to feel that there was a lot missing in their relationships. Some, more than others. I had read quite a lot about it, that it is common for people suffering from the challenges of epilepsy to also often have challenges and difficulties in their marriage.

But this was no excuse, more a reason to do so much more. To do so much more, because this was one issue which wasn't only missing, lost would be a better word to use. Both missing and lost. Lost because it simply couldn't find its way, like so many other parts of my life that had, over time, strengthened and recovered. Like some of those other values that had gradually become even better and stronger than they were prior to 2009.

But this was the one issue that was constantly pulling me down, constantly pulling me back. But worst of all, it was something I so dearly wanted and so dearly needed. Thus, it became so much heavier and so much more difficult to have it dragging behind me. What devastated me most was that we slept apart. Every evening was the same. I would leave; go away from the family, away from Bina, into that lonely dark corner of the house. This ritual had a large amount of meaning behind it. Well, at least for me it did. A meaning that had a great influence on me. You know what they say, "Actions speak louder than words".

One issue which I often thought about and often had me worried, was the close and special relationship I had with Sarah and Timmy. I was sure that they, especially Sarah, would eventually notice and feel the general mood at home and especially in the relationship between Bina and I as husband and wife.

I tried really hard to forget about myself and those missing pieces in my life. Especially when I was talking to people who I was meeting through the organisation and also elsewhere. In those instances when I put more emphasis on sharing words of optimism and confidence, when I knew I had to hide my weaknesses and pain. Doing this also helped me stay strong and confident and to stay content with life as it was.

Over time I kind of just left those that were to me lost parts of my life back there, giving them little or no attention or effort. I felt as if I had done everything I could. I felt this often enough when I tried to bring up the topic in conversation with Bina, but it only added more to the feeling that it was all going nowhere and that there was nothing more I could do.

But this wasn't something I could simply leave 'back there' and I certainly didn't want to. This wasn't a physical entity but entirely a psychological one, made up mostly of feelings, many individual pieces. Pieces I, as a human being, really needed. Pieces, which left this great emptiness inside of me. Emptiness I desperately wanted and needed to fill. Since I had become so much more emotional and sensitive, it only made it so much more difficult. So difficult and taxing, constantly pulling me back and dragging me and my feelings down, until it practically 'broke me'! But I almost allowed it to break away, because I didn't want this pulling me back and pulling me, my confidence, and my feelings down any longer. It was something I was going to have to let go of, if I was to progress any further. As I said earlier, I felt that I had done everything in my power and I felt that there was nothing more I could do.

What made it even sadder was how it affected me as a person. Of course, the first consequence was that over time I started to lose the feeling that I was someone's husband. But it didn't stop there. I gradually also started losing the feeling that I was even a man. And finally, and worst of all, when I started losing those feelings, I also started losing that feeling of pride that I was the father of my own children.

But it wasn't only at home and in my relationship with Bina where I felt like this. It was obviously there, where it struck the hardest. But it was also quite present outside and affected my social life too. What was true, and what made it even harder and why it affected me so much more, was that I was trying, trying really hard. Trying to make this connection with people in general, but so often it simply didn't work.

This made me think; "Is this the reason why so many people with epilepsy are so introvert, avoiding contact with people in general?" Nobody likes the feeling of rejection, so people continued living in their own solitary little world, avoiding contact with people. But I certainly didn't want this for myself, which is why I put a great deal of effort into avoiding it, almost right from the start.

So, what I started doing was searching for alternatives, to try and replace all these missing pieces. Additionally, life was constantly changing, which brought new adventures, new experiences and also new challenges, which I would otherwise never have experienced.

One day I noticed a caption about a local and well-known dating site on the internet, for people searching for new relationships. Even though I was having all these challenges and feelings of emptiness, which were constantly pulling me down, into this dark 'corner' of loneliness and sorrow, I never once thought of disrespecting or being unfaithful to Bina.

I always thought and always had it in my mind that these dating sites were exactly that, only dating sites, where people were looking for new relationships and partners. But when I saw how they emphasised that this site is for finding new contacts, new friends and, of course, new relationships, it attracted my attention and I decided to have a look, and even thought of maybe even trying it out. So, I did.

Going onto the site was quite foreign to me at first and I wasn't quite sure what to expect. I knew what I had set out to do, what my desires were. To find new friends, maybe someone with whom I could share my feelings, my emotions and for someone to show some of that respect I had gained etc. What I most wanted was to find a friend who could help bring back some of those things that I so dearly missed.

It didn't take long before I started expressing myself more easily with the ladies I was meeting and chatting to on the site. It was also interesting 'meeting' all these different people, from all different kinds of backgrounds.

As I started to express myself more freely, I made more connections with people. It didn't take long before I found individuals, who were in similar situations and facing similar challenges to me. I was building a circle of contacts.

There were a few individuals with whom I felt I was able to comfortably communicate and, at the same time, build a level of respect and trust. What was most special was to have that feeling of open two-way communication, which I so dearly missed.

It didn't take long before I found somebody with whom I could make a bit of a stronger connection. Her name was Andrea. We were both facing similar challenges and had feelings of emptiness in our relationships. Both of us also had quite similar views of life; respect for our children and fear of what separation could do to them, etc.

Andrea gave me the feeling that she was someone who would actually listen to me and, above all, someone who respected and showed compassion to my feelings too. I had somebody who allowed me to express myself, without the fear of unnecessary interruption. And I, with compassion and respect for her, listened to her too. These were those very valuable entities that I was yearning for. It slowly became a really special friendship.

I also admired her discipline and strength to keep our friendship going in the right direction. It was also because of this that our friendship grew and became really strong more than can be imagined. I had found exactly what I was looking for and exactly what my heart needed. Even though we mainly communicated through messages, e-mails and by phone, it was exactly what I so desperately needed.

We communicated often and were in regular contact. It was that two-way communication, that two-way relationship that I had been so desperately searching for. I was able to open up and share with her my feelings honestly, and so could she. We both found what we so longed for and what we were both looking for.

But our close friendship only lasted for so long. The fear of her husband finding out and the thought of what he could do to her was a constant burden on her mind. It wasn't until he started acting suspiciously, and also became more verbally abusive, that we agreed to stop our contact. It was a difficult decision to make. But it was a wise one and the correct one to make, for the both of us.

Andrea had shown me something special. The level of feelings I could feel in my heart for a person. Something I unfortunately was only feeling now for the first time in a really long time. Something which I honestly, sadly and unfortunately could not feel and was so desperately missing with Bina.

The period that followed was a really hard one for me and I eventually sunk back into a deep depression. Only this time, deeper than I had before. I was aware and it was obvious to me that I was going to sink back into that loneliness and darkness that I was in before I met Andrea.

But it was now even more difficult than I had ever expected it would be. Was it because of the level of respect and compassion I had gained for Andrea? Because I had once again felt and tasted the level and amount of feelings I could have and feel inside myself. You know how they say, "You only realise what you have once you lose it."

I tried to hide my sorrow and pain as much as I could and I tried really hard to keep my mind busy with other issues, but it was often just so pointless.

One of those issues I started putting more emphasis on and kept myself busy with, was with the work and tasks I was doing for the organisation for epilepsy, LIGA. The work and atmosphere of the work as a whole helped me strive to stay strong and optimistic, because I knew that people may need to rely on me for some positive support.

And that's exactly what happened. Something quite amazing, actually. It was quite sad but still an amazing coincidence. A lady who had come to the organisation barely two months before was inspired by what I had to say and felt comfortable with what I had shared with her, about her condition and about living with epilepsy. We remained in reasonably regular contact, chatting about various issues and challenges related to our conditions and also some of our personal experiences.

Then, one day she called me and I could hear her voice breaking up. At times she even found it difficult to talk. She had fallen into a depression, just like the experiences I was having. After she had eventually managed to explain what had triggered her to fall into this depressive state, I totally understood and felt exactly what she was going through.

She and her husband were experiencing quite a bit of friction in their relationship. It wasn't just arguments but the general atmosphere of their relationship, which had been dragging on for quite some time, which was bothering her. Pretty much like what I was going through. All she needed was somebody to talk to.

We had quite an lengthy discussion and she was really quite grateful that I listened and talked to her. I didn't really share any concrete information or opinions, as I had so many times before, when I had shared information or talked about epilepsy. All that was necessary was for the discussion to open up, for us to be able to openly talk about our individual issues, troubles and feelings. The discussion did a lot for me too, because we spoke about such big and relevant issues, those that were also bothering and troubling me. It opened up my mind and I found I could think about and face these issues a lot more easily, since I was no longer only thinking about my own issues, but I was now able to 'come out with them', knowing that I wasn't alone.

There were a few among the individuals that I was meeting with whom I developed good, unique and respectful friendships with. People who I could comfortably trust and share even the most personal issues. And now, even those issues, which until now I had been ignoring, hiding and constantly pushing aside.

There were certain individuals who showed me, directed me and guided me to confront my challenges. To be able to confront and take hold of those challenges, which I had been avoiding. The challenges I was not strong enough or confident enough to confront. But what was more valuable than opening up, and feeling more comfortable around people is that I was opening up more to myself.

It was one of those friends who helped me reach inside myself and helped pull out some of those attributes of being a man that I had practically lost and never regained. It was true that a portion of the great loneliness that I felt inside was the natural desire for sexual intercourse, which did eventually return after 2013. And since my relationship with Bina never recovered, I was constantly pushing it aside, feeling that it contradicted the respect that I had gained for women. The respect that I had gained for women was still totally dominating my mind and mentality.

The time had come for me to face and confront this challenge. Here I was, sitting with this one issue that was so often pulling me down, pulling me back into sadness and despair, while I was so confidently pushing forward and making such progress in so many other parts of life. It was a challenge that I wasn't confident enough or strong enough to confront.

But now I had this new friend. A person who had I met through the dating site. A person with whom I could build a special friendship. I noticed and felt her wisdom shortly after meeting her. This was someone with whom I could develop a really unique friendship, in the full and complete meaning of a friend. A special friend that I could feel was by my side as I confronted and faced this challenge. It was time for me to take hold of this one very serious and heavy issue. When I did eventually decide to take it on, I took it on as I had with so many other challenges in the past i.e. that I wouldn't let it go, but follow it to the end. "Either take care of it, or allow it to continue influencing and controlling my life".

On a number of occasions I had thought about what it would be like to leave, to separate and to move out and move on. Those few times when I had maybe talked with someone and when we chatted about the atmosphere of my relationship and the situation at home. They had suggested and recommended that a seperation would really be best, but I often disagreed and didn't want to listen and constantly pushed that aside. But now it was different, because now the decision had been made. It was time for me to do something about it.

That's how it remained in my mind, as something that was actually going to happen. It was no longer just an idea or suggestion that I didn't want to accept. The thoughts about what this really meant were now becoming so much deeper and more detailed. This was typical for me in many such situations, my thoughts would be really deep and down to detail. This time, also as deep as the seriousness of the issue itself.

But interestingly, as I started putting more and more emphasis and thought into moving away, all those feelings of progress and accomplishments I was making, slowly started melting away. Eventually this was the only thing I could and did think about. I started thinking more and more of what it all meant and what I would have to confront by moving away. And with time, the top of the hill, which was already so far away, almost totally disappeared. All I could see now was the journey.

This obviously greatly influenced my mood in general. Even the desire and enjoyment of cycling virtually disappeared. Even the enjoyment of going to work by bike and the refreshment it brought right at the beginning of each day was entirely gone. The appeal of taking relaxing walks through the town also faded. I still went for regular walks, though, but that's all they were, physical walks and nothing more. I was no longer getting that feeling that it was replenishing my body. I wondered whether this is what it feels like when a person falls into total depression.

It was quite interesting though, because all my feelings and emotions had practically disappeared. I had no satisfaction or enjoyment for anything. Virtually no feelings for anybody, sadly not even for my own children. OK that part is understandable, but at the same time there was no sadness, loneliness or emotional pain, nothing. I was simply a person, a being, practically lifeless. Many people around me noticed the difference. A couple of them asked me here and there what was wrong. But I obviously didn't say much.

While I was going through all of this, there was one very valuable thing I did have. It was the wisdom and friendship of that one lady I had met through the dating site. She stuck by me, even though I was at times so emotionally cold and with practically no desire to communicate or anything. It was totally clear to me that I had one person who understood me and what I was going through.

This emotional state also affected my physical wellbeing. It was more than just a lack of desire to do any cycling or physical activity. It also had an exceptionally great effect on my condition. I had two seizures, only about a week apart, which was utterly extraordinary and quite worrying. One of the seizures wasn't a full 'grand mal' seizure though, but I was conscious and pretty aware of myself and my actions. What I did remember was that I had very little orientation and was constantly bumping into things.

What followed the seizures and became even more worrying was my memory. I had difficulty 'taking in' and remembering small bits of information, relating to minor and more insignificant tasks. I didn't have as much difficulty with larger tasks and those with more important amounts of information, which required more concentration. It was quite annoying because it influenced me practically everywhere, from my responsibilities at work, to chatting with people.

The problem with my memory eased off and got a lot better as soon as I went through the emotional side of the separation. This was a clear indication of why this was happening to me in the first place, as well as being an indication of how great and emotional this step was for me.

I was already quite interested in the effects of psychological wellbeing on epilepsy and epileptic seizures. So I assumed right away, as soon as it all got better, that the emotional stress was to blame for the seizures and difficulties I was having with my memory.

In my opinion, this was the greatest and most emotionally challenging situation I had ever found myself in. It was during this time that I also 'tasted' and felt the true and full meaning of what a real friend is. From the few individuals who stuck by my side the whole time and who at times had to even push me to keep me going.

What Andrea and some of the other special friends I had made showed me, were the true values of a good friendship. And especially confirmed that my intentions and aspirations by going onto the site were in no way exaggerated or wrong, considering the situation I had found myself in. Rather they were entirely realistic and something other people were also experiencing, searching for and doing. These friends fulfilled that valuable feeling of being accepted.

What this was actually showing me, or rather what was happening to me, was that I was changing. It was because of me changing, that I started to take more notice of these new friends. I always had a group of friends and acquaintances, but having any of those unique or special friends was something almost nonexistent.

I like what young opera singer Jonathan Antoine said, when he described the experiences he had with depression. He said, "I had a descent group of friends. But I wasn't confident in myself; I didn't like myself, which made that group of friends 'null and void', because you can't like anyone, if you don't like yourself."

That is so true what he said. The feelings I had, for these new friends were all a part of this journey I was on in finding myself.

My feelings about myself and also my natural desire for sexual intercourse also slowly changed. From my point of view, there were two main reasons for this. I was slowly returning to becoming a man because I was no longer pushing those emotions aside during the challenges I was having with Bina. And secondly, because I had the feeling of having special people in my life again.

Well that is it, another chapter of experiences! When at first, and for quite some time, I didn't really want to accept or welcome people into my life, and also moments when I simply didn't want anyone there. It was totally understandable that I lost a number of friends because of it, because "who wants to be with a person like that". But when you try to recover from something like this, the desire, the need, to feel accepted and loved becomes really big. That's something which has given me and also shown me, the respect and gratitude of what a true friend really is. Something which made it possible to create the unique friendships that I was now able to make and have in my life.

Well that's the person I am becoming. I've already mentioned a number of times the respect I gained for people and their feelings, especially during and after my recovery, after the incident of December 2008 and later, with all that I have experienced. That's mainly because I am quite emotional and my feelings are sensitive and valuable. A greater part of my feelings and emotions is to love and be loved.

If there was only one thing that all these challenges and experiences were doing for me, it was that they were opening me up in different directions. I was actually meeting more different people. I was becoming more comfortable talking to people about all kinds of things. Basically, it was another great step in 'getting out' and opening up more.

Chapter fifteen

We've all had it happen. You create something and when you have a look at what you have in your hands, or you look back at it you say to yourself: "WOW! Did I do that?"

Well these kind of things also quite often happened to me. As I was pushing forward, moving onwards and upwards, higher and higher, along the road of life. I stopped a couple of times to have a look back and to see where I was and ended up saying to myself, "Look how far I've come, all the way up to here! SO HIGH!" But still, as I turn back around and look forward, I see, I still need to carry on.

Not far from my hometown Kamnik, there is a hill, well-known by practically all cyclists. The road winds through the hills, up the side of one mountain and over a mountain pass. At the top, there is a well-known pub and cottage called the 902. It is at the peak of the pass, at 902 metres above sea-level. To get there, you don't need to go far out of town before the incline starts. There are some really challenging stages as the road snakes its way up the hillside. In some places the road has such sharp hairpin bends that it virtually doubles back on itself as it snakes its way up the side of the mountain. Then there are stages where the road actually goes a little downhill. Imagine going up there for the first time. You're not familiar with the route and you don't know what is waiting for you around the next bend. You don't even know how far you have to go. Then, all of a sudden, a break in the vegetation alongside the road and in front of you, is the '902'. You've made it to the top!

I'm sure a lot of people who aren't so physically active, who see these cyclists going up roads like the one up to the '902', say to themselves, "These guys are crazy! What do they see in this?"

When I decide to go cycling, I often ponder, “Where should I go today?” I could simply choose an easy route on flat terrain, which I often do. But I don’t get the same satisfaction out of it as I do when I take on a more challenging one, such as to the ‘902’. Summers in Kamnik are really nice. There are always many cyclists going out willingly, enjoying their chosen challenges, knowing what each challenge brings them.

Life is so much like cycling. It could be like a route on flat terrain, or even downhill. Nice and easy, irrelevant of how long it is. Or it could be a more challenging one like one snaking its way up the side of a mountain. With bends and challenging slopes of different kinds, and you not knowing what lies around the next bend

That’s how it was often for me as I was pushing my way forward along the road of life. Not knowing how steep it’s going to be around the next bend, or how many more bends there are still waiting for me. But, as I look back, it brings me satisfaction, remembering and seeing what I’ve been through and to actually see how far I have in fact come.

What sometimes also helps me strive and keep pushing forward is where I live - Slovenia. Even though Slovenia has been independent for around 25 years, independent from socialist rule, the socialist attitude is still so present in the people. They are so used to doing everything by the book, according to some rule or instruction, and one can easily see where it’s getting them. This only gives me more encouragement to put that much more emphasis on what I can do, for my own wellbeing, or for anything else, as a matter of a fact. Instead of just sitting around and waiting for instructions or solutions.

Another characteristic that is so evident in Slovenes is their pessimism. I don’t know if this has anything to do with the socialist rule the country was under in the past, but what it has helped me realise, is the value of optimism.

These two factors have greatly helped and guided me to turn the problem of having to live with epilepsy into a challenge. Thus, into a way of life where epilepsy is a part of life and not a gate restricting it.

As I look back at the past, I can gladly and proudly say to myself, "Yes, I have, I've made it up to here, to a height I have never been before."

When I look back at what I've been through and what I've achieved, I sometimes say to myself, "How did I do this? I couldn't have done all this on my own", and I didn't. It was those friends, whose friendship was more than just somebody you know or somebody you spend some free time with every now and then at the local pub. It's those friends who stay by your side as you travel along the routes of life. It's those friends who stick by your side as you hit the steepest slopes, and if necessary even help you climb them.

Interestingly, here is another situation where life experiences can be closely compared to cycling. If you decide to go up to the '902', or any cycling challenge with a friend, you'll notice that you are able to do it at a faster pace and more easily than you are normally able to do on your own. And when you get to the top, you quickly notice how you managed it a lot easier too, compared to when you go alone. Thus, quicker and easier. Is it because your friend subconsciously 'pushes you' that much more? I don't know. You might even find out that you are actually able to do it a lot quicker and easier than you thought. All you needed was for your friend to show you that you are better and more capable than you thought you were.

The only difference between cycling and real life is that in cycling, you almost always end up where you began. In life it would be best if you could always stay at the top. But that is unfortunately normally impossible and unreal. There are days or periods when you feel you are at the peak. Then, soon afterwards, you find yourself back at the base.

There was one such instance, when I had that feeling as if I was back at the base, or even lower, when one of my friends stepped up and recommended something. He said that if I have a memory of an event or a time when I felt lifted up and strong, and if I can remember where that took place, "Go back to that place, and just be there, it will lift you back up and you'll find your strength again".

What came to mind was the time, the moment at the train station, when I decided that I was not going to allow this condition to take me over. That was one really big event that I won't easily forget.

Then, not long after, I shared this with another friend. An even closer friend. What she added to this was really wise and so true. She said, "Are you still back there, or are you better than you were on that day?". A really wise reaction and something valuable to remember. She added, "Even though you might feel as if absolutely everything is going wrong, remember, you are still a lot further than you were back on that day".

For me it means a lot if I can simply feel and consider myself at a higher point than I was in the past. That is enough to keep me pushing forward and something my friends were also giving me.

I have had a number of experiences where my friends have helped me reach new heights and showed me what I am really capable of.

One such unique friendship was the one that emerged from helping the two foreigners at the bread counter in the grocery store which, in turn, led me to find another foreigner living here in Kamnik, Noah Charney. We were in quite regular contact with each other and our friendship grew quite quickly. It didn't take long before we were chatting about what we do and where our interests lie, and so on.

One of Noahs' main interests is writing. He has also taken it quite far and it has become a great part of his profession. He writes a lot of articles for a number of leading journals around the world. He has also written a couple of novels, which have become well known and which have given him a name in writing. He holds classes in writing, teaching people the basics about writing. In conclusion, he's quite an active writer.

I continued sharing with him more of the experiences I was going through regarding epilepsy, and also a bit about my personal life. He found it really quite intriguing and interesting and concluded that I had quite a story to tell, which would make interesting reading. He then mentioned and invited me to come to some of his workshops, where he spoke and taught some of the basics about writing. So that's what I did.

I had always been a little interested in writing, so this new encouragement only added to that interest, and provided me with additional enthusiasm and encouraged me to start writing "my story". As time went on, and as we spoke more and more about writing, I became even more inspired to start writing, so I did.

But it wasn't only about writing "My story". As I thought about it, I became inspired to write about one big event in my life, which I thought could also make interesting reading - taking part in my first ever cycling marathon. I wrote about all the concerns, preparations and considerations, which were involved as a person suffering from epilepsy taking part in competitive sports. I sent my article to an Australian website, which gladly accepted and published it. I also sent a Slovene translation to the epilepsy organisation in Slovenia, so it was published in their journal for epilepsy too.

This is another good example of what a good friend and friendship can do for a person it showed the value and importance of having people around you. It really lifted my self-esteem higher and pulled out and amplified another hidden talent to a level it never been. Something I would never have achieved by myself.

It also showed how something quite insignificant, like deciding to help somebody in a grocery store, can do and what can come out of it. Obviously, there is a great deal involved, for this to have come so far. I think first and foremost, how I can comfortably and easily confront and open up to strangers. When I got to know Noah a bit better, it made for open conversation, while at the same time I allowed myself to change. One very important component, important at every step, is the optimism on which I was constantly putting special emphasis.

Life goes on. I have become really appreciative of life and take more notice of what goes on around me. I often ponder how life would have turned out if the event of December 2008 hadn't have happened, and, of course, everything that subsequently followed because of it. One thing is for sure, I for certainly wouldn't have met some of the amazing people I have met along the way.

Chapter sixteen

Well, here I am. Eight years after my brain, mind, and practically my entire body, took that crash and hit the reset button. Just like a computer system which crashed and needed to be restarted, some data and contents were lost and needed to be replaced.

I'm sure you've all heard, or even said, to yourselves, "Oh, if only I had a reset button, so I could start all over again". In many ways, I really feel like that is what happened to me. During the incident of December 2008, my complete system crashed and, to a great extent, restarted itself.

Today I look back and see with what my memory has been 'filled'. Not only with what, but also when, how and why it all filled up and became like it is today.

One of the greatest blessings is that I started off with almost nothing; no feelings, a changed mentality, very little memory and, as I have repeated over and over again, no feelings. You certainly must be asking yourself, "How on earth can he see this as a blessing?"

Yes, it really was an unimaginable and horrible experience. Something I would never want anyone to have to go through. It was an extraordinary challenge getting myself back to where I am today. I really lost a great deal because of it and the journey to completely (re)find myself is still not quite finished. But what this journey and all these experiences have given me, is an amazing appreciation and respect for all that I have.

Additionally, what I have been through has given me an understanding and respect for those people who are facing health conditions, whatever they may be.

If there was one thing I could give people who have to go through challenges such as having to live with epilepsy or any other similar condition, it is the capacity to understand.

The first thing for each and every individual who is living with such a condition and the daily challenges it brings, is for them to understand the condition. With understanding, comes acceptance. Through acceptance you are able to practically take the condition by the hand and together with it, move forward in life.

The second piece of understanding is directed at those who are in close or regular contact with anyone facing such a condition, in other words: family members, relatives, friends, ..., everybody. It is important that they understand and accept that this person is different, irrespective of how normal they may seem, or how insignificant the condition may seem. Remember, they have this condition all the time. Wherever they go and whatever they may be doing, it goes with them and is with them the whole time. For each and every individual it is different and it affects each person differently.

My interest and curiosity in living with, understanding, and surviving epilepsy will never end. And I am applying the same effort and curiosity into what I am doing to help others living with the condition.

One instance I will never forget is when I was talking with one of the leading neurologists in Slovenia, during which I mentioned my interest in studying epilepsy and in assisting others suffering from it. I mentioned how I constantly ask myself, "How far can I go in helping others, I am not a doctor or a specialist?" It was his reaction which made a big impression. He said that I have something that no specialist or doctor has, and that is experience. I have something which unites me with people, which is understanding, and thus the ability to empathise with what it is like living with such a condition.

Some of the examples of what other well-known and famous people have done and how far they have taken their challenges is something which also gives me that extra courage to keep pushing forward and keep moving. People like Tony Greig, a cricket legend and commentator, who didn't allow epilepsy to stop him and thus became a renowned cricket player and later a world reknowned commentator of the sport. And another, the singer, Ronan Keating, although not suffering from epilepsy, went through many challenges associated with illness and what illness brings to become the person he is now. This is just an example of two people who stood up to the challenges life threw at them, and by speaking out they became ambassadors and defeated their challenges.

It is my choice which route I am going to take and follow. And one of the routes is to learn. Learn from what has happened to me, from my individual experiences and, in so doing, continue forward on my journey to becoming the best person I possibly can.

I know that 'Bina' didn't really like me sharing my story, and has sometimes expressed her disapproval' She doesn't like the fact that I am sharing some details about my personal life and I understand her. I know I am far from perfect, I know I have tripped and fallen over many challenges. But **I live a life I am not ashamed to talk about**.

It's with this attitude that I have managed to reach some of my greatest achievements, one of which was to be able to successfully compete in a competitive sport.

I'd like to conclude with how and why I succeeded. It's because I wanted to. I simply took all the possible steps and precautions to be able to successfully and proudly do this, and importantly, I did, I succeeded. The reason: **because I wanted to**.

ABOUT THE AUTHOR

In his childhood, Robert lived in South Africa. At the age of 20, he moved to Slovenia, where he continued his studies in engineering.
With the introduction of epilepsy into his life, and after facing the many challenges of having epilepsy, Robert's interest in living with and challenging epilepsy grew. Robert has written a number of articles about living an active life, while facing the challenges of living with epilepsy.
He is also very active in sports and puts extra emphasis on being able to live a physically active life alongside having epilepsy. Robert has also studied and written a number of articles about taking part in competitive sports.

20323096R00070

Printed in Great Britain
by Amazon